JOE E.R.

JOE E.R.

Hospital Volunteer

Joe Apple

March, 2019

EARTHQUAKES AND VOLCANOES

I t was my first night in the ER and I think I was just as scared as the pale, white-haired grandmother that had just been rolled in by paramedics.

She was the first of many I was to see over the next eleven years during my Saturday nights as a volunteer in the emergency room from 8:00 PM to midnight.

Her eyes were half-closed with mouth gaping open, taking quick, short gasps of air. With dentures removed, her mouth resembled a mud volcano I once saw in the desert by the Salton Sea. Only, instead of mud spurting out, there was this pink, frothy liquid that reminded me of bubbles from a child's bubble bath.

Her blue and white cotton nightgown with the small pink flowers gave evidence of having been transported straight from bed.

Some came from nursing homes while others would be transported from the residence they had occupied for many years. An artery would get plugged or something would *blow*, and here they would be brought.

I was reminded of the movie, "Soylent Green," starring Charlton Heston as he discovered the world's food supply consisted of *reprocessed* people. The deceased would be rolled to a room on gur-

Joseph Apple

neys, stuffed into bags and loaded onto trucks.

Fortunately, we don't do that these days (I think).

We have a memorial service to pay tribute to their short time here on earth, then shove 'em back into the ground...from which *Adam* came.

From my training, I suspected her heart was giving out and fluid was backing up into her lungs. The triage nurse quickly guided her into a *stall*, but not with the speed of rushing to a house-fire with screaming children upstairs. Instead, it looked like she was pushing a shopping cart to a register that had just opened at Target.

The pale grandmother would be *gone* by morning. But I would have no way of knowing that just yet. I would seldom learn what happened to ER patients once they were rolled down the corridor to the elevator.

Hopefully, my fears concerning *green*, St. Patrick's Day breakfast bars will never be substantiated.

As an automobile mechanic at a private university, I was allowed the benefit of taking two classes each semester, tuition-free. I was branching out in an attempt to learn what I might be able to do in the world of medicine.

One day three nurses from a local hospital came to my anatomy class looking for volunteers...usually getting nursing students. This was a good way to discover if you were cut out for a life of medical service.

Several students would learn the hard way that they could not stand to be around real, live patients...and occasionally a dead one.

My *escort* from Family Services, Julia, with the short black hair that reminded me of a *ducktail* cut from the sixties, seemed uncomfortable to be here herself. She was clad in a dark blue, knee-length skirt with closely-tailored matching jacket and white polyester chiffon blouse with the high neck.

She sported a look of complete calmness that would have sobered even the most belligerent drunk. Or, maybe we were about to board a Delta airliner for France?

She whispered under her breath the ER staff never enjoyed seeing her here, since that usually meant a patient or family member had complained about a lost shoe, or a mother's blackened arm from multiple IV stab attempts.

For some sick reason, I recalled an old "Mommy, Mommy" joke from my youth.

"Mommy, Mommy...Daddy has a bruise on his arm!"

"Shut up Johnny and eat around it!"

I wasn't feeling very good about this.

As an older adult, the presumption was made that I might be a more *mature* volunteer and able to handle the fast-paced demands of a busy, full-trauma Emergency Department.

Notice I used the word, *presumption*.

I always wanted to work somewhere in medicine...which usually implied you were up to speed in your math, science and chemistry.

Like my dad, I was a decent automobile mechanic and knew my way around carburetors, injectors and tapered roller wheel bearings. But being the fourth of ten kids from a small Indiana town was not the ideal platform from which to launch such an operation.

I figured high school was the place to identify those subjects I would want to avoid later in life...like...History, Spanish, Algebra and a few others.

After school, I only wanted to rush into the woods and sneak up on muskrats playing in the water. Instead, I always had that afternoon paper route to wear me down.

Money was hard to come by, and the cardboard in the bottoms of my shoes kept reminding me where I stood.

Julia said she had to go, and that I was on my own to see if I could make this thing work.

I had been given a copy of a similar plan, developed at Stanford University Hospital for a volunteer, patient-liaison position in the ER. But I did not know anyone in this ER and was not sure what I was even allowed to do.

If Julia, a for-real employee, was scared to be here, what chance did I have?

My document said I should talk to patients in the waiting room to comfort them and keep them informed concerning their loved ones. But I was more frightened than they were, and had no clue about their loved ones.

The sick and injured would be in the middle of blood tests, X-rays, cultures and urine analysis. Even the doctor often would not know what was going on until the lab results came in.

How was I to handle all these real-life, grown-up questions...me, the automobile mechanic with the C- in chemistry?

I later learned that the staff considered the waiting room to be a no-man's land that should be avoided at all costs! Even the most seasoned nurse avoided going *out there*!

I wanted to put up my best front, so I wore my dark blue slacks with cuffs and pleats in front...long sleeve pin-striped shirt and burgundy tie with off-white diamonds...black shoes and dark blue socks with red, cross-hatched lines.

I thought I looked very official.

I sported a photo ID clipped to one lapel of my light blue, volunteer jacket with patches that identified me as an *official volunteer.* I also carried a clipboard with my notes and diagrams of the hospital layout.

My *notes* consisted of door codes so I wouldn't get locked outside the building, and names of nurses I was trying to memorize, with descriptions...

Becky...dishwater blonde hair...fat legs and grumpy.

But to be fair, I learned it didn't take much to become grumpy in there...at the end of a twelve-hour shift...three drunks from a Dodger's game and one sleepy homeless guy who would take a swing at her if she attempted to insert an IV in his neck (the only viable vein left).

Everyone was rushing around, doing their jobs. I learned that no one had the time or inclination to answer dumb questions.

"Where are the full oxygen bottles kept?"

"I don't know...somewhere down the hall in one of those closets...go ask someone down there."

I was afraid to ask questions or do anything for fear I might do the wrong thing. So for four Saturday nights, I manned my post at the hallway entrance, clipboard in hand, making notes to myself...

Diane...mole on left cheek...man-hands...grumpy.

And then something fortuitous happened. As I was vacating my post at midnight on that fourth Saturday, *Billie*, with the red pony-tail, braces and large breasts, happened to mention that they could *finally* relax, now that I was leaving.

I quickly realized they thought I had been *planted* there by the front office to spy on them.

Off came the tie, *out* went the nice shirt, *bye-bye* clipboard.

I bought a pair of burgundy scrubs and white tennis shoes to go with the blue volunteer jacket. I was determined to just start *doing* things, and then see if I got yelled at.

Mind you, I was not about to start pulling IV's or adjusting oxygen valves, but surely I could clean up messy gurneys, change linens and learn where all the supplies were kept.

The *fine print* in my volunteer information packet said volunteers would not be subjected to blood and bodily fluids. But I doubt the author of that document foresaw the jungle pathway I was hacking with my machete.

I decided to start cleaning up messes...something I could surely do on my own.

I had the brains to wear gloves, which there were plenty of. I kept one pocket of my blue volunteer jacket stuffed with large, size ten, purple gloves of which I would go through many pairs before midnight.

I picked my first gurney to clean.

It took a while to learn all the small details when wondering if a patient was *gone*, or had only limped down a hallway to use the restroom.

If the patient's blood-stained jeans were stuffed into a plastic patient-belongings bag with sandals, blue t-shirt and white Jockey underwear, it was a good bet they were still around somewhere... but not always.

I could ask a nurse, but I soon learned every nurse had his or her own *three beds* to cover, and the nurse I needed to talk to was *never* there just then. And none of the other nurses knew exactly who was covering which beds. A chart on the wall was supposed to explain *who,* had *which* beds. But you could never be sure.

As I would often have to do, I just jumped in and began *swimming,* or, dog-paddling. I wasn't in over my head yet, so if necessary, I could always paddle to one side and climb out.

All the *signs* seemed in order:

The cover-sheet and blanket were rolled into a heap...a half-empty IV bag of saline solution with capped end was hanging on its pole...a couple of heart monitor sticky-tabs were stuck to the sheet...a used bottle of sterile saline solution and hydrogen peroxide were sitting on the bedside cabinet...and small blood stains were evident about where I would expect a pair of knees to rest with dirt and gravel all around.

I felt like I was playing *Clue*...was it the *butler* in the *pantry* with the *candlestick?*

Nope, it was a *mid-forties male* on the *sidewalk* with a *skateboard.*

Since there were only *small* blood stains, I wasn't sure if the sheet needed to be dumped into the *red* bucket reserved for blood-stained articles.

At first, I began putting anything *suspected* into the *red can.* But I soon realized there were *stages* of contamination. Besides, the red can could not possibly hold all the minor blood-stained articles I was to run across.

I decided this sheet was going into the regular dirty-clothes hamper. I looked over my shoulder to see if I was going to get yelled at, but no one seemed to be complaining.

One small step for the volunteer, one giant leap for mankind.

I knew that everything needed to be wiped down and sterilized before applying the clean sheet, so I proceeded to do so with a sanitized *wipe.*

The *wipes* were long, connected, heavy-duty paper towels that had been soaked in an anti-bacterial solution inside the round, green-and-white plastic container hanging on the wall (Green and

Joseph Apple

white seemed to be favorite colors in the ER).

The *paper towels* protruding from the top of the canister looked like miniature bed sheets being forced out the top of a volcano.

For some reason, everything in the ER reminded me of volcanoes and earthquakes.

Since the wipes were supposed to sanitize the bed, I thought I could use my bare hands...you know, like this might be good for my hands as well? But nurse A, whose gurney I was cleaning, stepped in and advised me I should wear gloves when handling the wipes. She said the wipes contained hazardous chemicals with known carcinogens.

I thought that odd. Things that *sanitize* also kill people.

There seemed to be a fine line between *cleaning* and *killing*. I guess it all depended on which side of the microbial bacteria line you found yourself on. In any event, the cleaning agents seemed to pose more risks for me than the germy gurney, so I pulled out the gloves.

Nurse A *corrected* me, but did not actually *yell* at me, so that was progress. I was invading her territory by stepping in and cleaning *her* gurney, but I think she was beginning to see the benefit in this...like, less work for her?

In the future, only the new kids (they all looked like kids) would get edgy when I invaded their turf. But they all soon realized I could vastly improve the quality of their work-lives.

All that was necessary now was for me to figure out what I was doing? And then, in stepped nurse B. She saved my life in the ER.

Nurse B stood around 5' 4"... was shaped like a bowling pin with scraggly, medium-length, brown hair and a face like a mud fence. But she was very outgoing and latched on to me. Being a 50's-guy, my only guess was that she was in need of a strong father-figure.

I sincerely hoped she did not have the *hots* for me.

I had already learned that when a young female showed a strong interest in me, I should cover my wallet with one hand and start looking around for her *accomplice*.

For whatever reason, she was very friendly towards me and began showing me the ropes. This was exactly the person I was *praying* for (except for possibly the face).

She explained that some nurses *doubled* the sheet when making up a gurney, since that looked neater. But when transferring a patient from gurney-to-bed via the sheet alone, the thing needed to be opened and in one layer in order to safely grasp and transfer the patient from said gurney-to-bed without dropping them in a heap on the floor.

I quickly removed my sheet and un-folded the thing.

I looked at my first bed and felt very proud of myself. It looked neat and professional. Now it was time to start talking to patients.

I was warned to always introduce myself as a *volunteer* to avoid someone thinking I might be the doctor. Some people could be deficient in their English skills and might not be able to read the large *VOLUNTEER* patch on my jacket.

NO-MAN'S LAND

The Waiting Room

L ooking out from the inside, the waiting room seemed like a zoo. Only, I was on the *inside* and behind the laminated safety glass that protected *me* from *them*.

Maybe this is how apes at the zoo feel when looking at all the visitors streaming by? But which one was I...ape?, or vacationer from Arizona? When comparing the *outside* to the *inside*, I found it a tough call as to *who* was *who*?

I could see a 50's-gal in one corner wearing a purple and yellow cotton blouse, gray sweat pants, no bra, flip-flops and holding a blue and white checked cotton dish towel to her head. There did not seem to be any blood, but she was obviously in great pain.

...all the indications of a full-blown migraine.

In the center sat a 30's Hispanic mom with two toddlers tugging at a copy of a four-year-old Newsweek magazine. No one had a white identification band applied to their wrist, so I assumed she was waiting for a family member on *my side...whichever side this was?*

In another corner sat a lone female teenager wearing a red, low-cut top and tight low-waist Levis. She already had her I.D. band on right wrist. There were no obvious signs to go by, so I had no clue why she was here.

In another corner sat/stood four African-American young people...males and females, obviously agitated and arguing loudly.

One male seemed to be angrier than the rest. He was wearing a nicely tailored black, long-sleeved silk shirt. The top buttons were open with several gold chains visible. His shiny, black, wavy hair was neatly styled, in contrast to his angry demeanor.

I could not yet hear what they were saying, but something seemed to be amiss in *Dodge City.*
The waiting room was originally intended to hold an appropriate number of people matching the size of the ten-bed ER.

With expansion to now over thirty beds, the waiting room was often packed to overflowing with even more people outside on park benches.

The color TV, with volume-control knob removed was mounted high in one corner of the room.

The Dodgers were playing the Angels tonight.

I could only guess at how many were actually interested in the game. Its purpose was not to *entertain*, but to *distract*. The game was being televised, so it must have been a sellout...which meant more drunks later.

I hesitated going out there (okay, it's *out there*), knowing I would be of limited help. But somehow, my going out there seemed to be helpful to some. I guess they viewed it as someone from *the inside* coming out to the trenches where *they* were huddled.

I tried to talk myself out of it, but there was nothing else for me to do just then...I was wracking my brain for *something...anything*. All the gurneys were made and there were no big messes to clean up.

Okay, here I go.

And so, after a final deep breath, I strode out to the Mexican mom with the two toddlers. I wanted to start with possibly the easiest...maybe she spoke no English at all? I know a little Spanish, but would probably get myself into big trouble.

"Mi Espanol es muy petite."

See?

I tried standing tall with no slouching. *Slouching* would give me away, I thought.

I did not want to display any fear.

I also did not want them to see the Mambo dance my knees were doing.

I wished there was a book at Borders for do-it-yourself lion tamers I could have studied before-hand...or one of those black-and-yellow, "Lion-Taming for Idiots" books?

At home, I rehearsed what I planned to say in front of our full-length mirror on the back of the bathroom door.

I hoped I could remember it properly:

"Hi, I'm Joe from *Patient Services* (a title I made up) and would just like to know if everything was going okay out here?"

Of course, *everything* was NOT okay, and hence the reason for being in the emergency room. And I already knew that. But those words often led to a response I could elaborate on.

As it turned out, she spoke perfect English (rats) and came from an affluent neighborhood.

If they began asking detailed medical questions concerning their loved ones, I then quickly made sure they knew I was a *volunteer* and would not have those answers. Although, once in a while I knew.

If a biker came in with one leg over a shoulder, I could *guess* (It had happened).

My job was to put people at ease without having all the answers... or *any* of the answers. To know what I was looking at, I would ask if they were with a patient on the inside, or waiting themselves to be seen?

She was waiting to hear about her husband who had experienced chest pains after shoveling dirt around the new Jacuzzi. He wanted to save as much as possible on the job.

I understood that. My wife had taught me how to pinch pennies as well.

And this information told me something about her. I knew to be very straight with her and not fool around. I could envision her going straight to the ER supervisor if she was not happy with my performance.

After going through the process several times of bugging the nurses about letting family come back, I learned how it worked.

It would be okay to bring family back after the initial work had been completed, which involved EKG* chest leads hooked up, *vitals* gathered, clothes off and into one of those backless gowns that all the patients loved so much. This usually took about fifteen minutes.

EKG (electrocardiogram), a heart scan, had been changed to *ECG*, which sounded too much like *EEG* (electroencephalogram), a brain scan, and so it is now back to *EKG* in most circles.

Once I got used to this routine, I would take matters into my own hands and actually do something on my own, which made me feel pretty important.

The door into the *business-part* of the ER from the waiting room was a *secure* door with a ten-button key pad. I had been given the code, which also elevated my status.

You know, I am important!

After disappearing into the ER and now back, I held the door open and motioned to the Mexican wife to follow me. The others in the waiting room would see this take place, and so my level of authority greatly enhanced.

I felt like a lion tamer who had fooled one lion into jumping on top of a big stand.

I was feeling braver all the time.

But suddenly, I remembered small children were not allowed to be with patients. That is not a stab against kids, it is just that they are more likely to harbor contagious viruses we all catch as kids.

We hurriedly worked it out. I would quickly escort the gal to her husband's bedside and return to babysit the kids...oh joy! My favorite nurse, *Miss Mud Face,* had already shown me where the comic books, crayons and stickers were kept...second drawer on the left, next to the sink.

Entertaining kids in a strange, new setting without their parents was always a tricky exercise. I felt like I was photographing great white sharks from inside an iron bar cage that was approved for *sea lions only.*

I dangled the comic books in front of them, carefully watching their reactions. To my relief, they lurched for them (and shook vigorously).

All I needed to do from then on was make sure they had their favorite colors. After pasting stickers on *both* best colorings, I was home free.

To my relief, the mother was soon back. Like any good mom, she did not want to leave her kids too long with the stranger.

Her husband would be kept for a while as his heart was moni-tored. Blood samples would be drawn as well, checking for spe-cial proteins that might offer clues to a possible *infarction*... an-other cool word for heart attack.

Okay, that was one successful move on my part.

Now...on to the young gal in the red, low-cut top.

I am sure she heard my *spiel* as I introduced myself to the Mexican mom. But I wanted to deliver all my comments to each person as though *they* were the only one in the room. I am sure it helped to make things more personal.

She did not want to talk, but asked how long it might be? When I was brand new at this I never had a good answer for that question. And no one ever knows for sure.

It's an impossible question to answer.

An elderly man suffering from a stroke could be rolled in at any moment, commanding the attention of half the staff.

After a while I learned to judge for myself how long they would be sitting. The rule was:

"Those closest to dying would be seen first."

No one liked hearing that from me (and I seldom said it), but that was the best answer.

In her case, I knew her wait would be long. She did not seem to be in great pain, and a long way from death. I never asked why people came to the ER, but she let it slip that she thought she was preg-nant, and things did not seem right.

I was not about to ask about *bleeding* or anything personal. So I told her it would be about two hours (or longer) and that she should be prepared for a wait.

The triage nurse had already checked her in and had her on the list. But as I told everyone, if their symptoms were to change and they suddenly felt worse, they were to buzz the triage nurse again. That helped give them the *sensation* they had some control over their situation.

Okay, two down and two to go.

I next moved on to the middle-aged gal with the blue dish towel to her head.

From the tears in her eyes and the awful grimace on her face, I decided to skip my introductory remarks and just asked how she was feeling? As I had suspected, she did indeed have a history of migraine headaches. I knew their would be little anyone could do for her, and that she would be one of the last to be seen.

Unfortunately for her, she was in one of the worst places she could possibly be.

Four young people were arguing and fighting over the length of the wait, making a lot of noise. Of course, this was doing wonders for the *migraine*.

Those making all the noise had just come from a party. I didn't really have to introduce myself. The loudest of the foursome jumped on me and asked why their friend had not immediately been given a room? I used my best golden-tone voice as I assured them the injured party would be seen in due fashion.

Mr. Loudmouth (with alcohol on his breath) then explained to me that their friend might have serious eye damage from a wine-bottle cork that had popped up, hitting her in the eye. I wanted to laugh, but could hear every sensible neuron in my brain screaming, "Don't do it!"

He yelled that if they had to wait longer than fifteen minutes, then they might go somewhere else. I did not have to think long about this one, as I told him the wait would be *at least* four hours.

I was worried about the poor gal with the migraine.

She couldn't take it any longer and ran outside. The *scratched eyeball* and company then decided to hit the road, which did not disappoint anyone.

I wanted to console the *migraine*, but she was better off out there by herself.

I probably was not supposed to do this, but I got a warm blanket from the heater and placed on her lap as she sat on the green, wooden bench outside. It would be a long and torturous night for her.

I thought I was finished with making my *rounds* when a heavy-set gal tried making it through the doorway and into the waiting room. Instead, she collapsed onto the floor, with the automatic door bumping into her ample *buttocks* (a real medical term), over and over.

I quickly entered my door code and alerted the triage nurse to the situation. As I bent over her, she began puking her guts out, all over the light green, vinyl flooring.

It was a "beer puke."

She was wearing a blue and white, cotton, number 99, *Manny Ramirez* baseball jersey.

Oh yeah...the Dodgers vs. Angels game. I had forgotten.

A beer-puke is not your ordinary puke. It has its own characteristic look, smell and feel. It normally has a light yellow color.

I could see large chunks of undigested nachos and cheese.

The cheese gave the normally light yellow beer-color more depth, and a velvety rich sheen. Some of the chip-fragments looked almost good enough to eat again...

...*almost.*

But the smell was still the same... like a port-a-potty outside a

Budweiser Bowling Bash.

I doubted she was being scouted for Manny's fan club.

A gurney was rapidly wheeled around, the gal loaded, and whisked inside. It then occurred to me how a patient might go about getting a bed quickly?

In the future, I would use this example to explain to new patients how to avoid the wait. If they had the nerve, all they needed to do was walk to the door and drop to the floor.

Puking is a nice touch, but won't gain you any friends... *housekeeping!!*

So far, no one (thankfully) has taken me up on the advice. But it *will* work.

THE BUILDING PROPER

T he emergency room had been expanded several times, so it took me a while to learn how to get around.

I was confused as to why some patients would be escorted out a second door on the far side of the waiting room. I did not realize that particular door led into ER II. We had seven sections if you included the hallways.

ER's V, VI, and VII were single beds in corridors, and great places to put the drunks.

I did not want to be embarrassed, so it was a while before I ventured to that other door on the far side of the waiting room to see if my door code would also work over there (It didn't). So I avoided using that door at all costs.

I had been doing this long enough that everyone assumed I knew the door codes, so it was too late to ask.

It was like meeting a seldom-seen co-worker whose name I had never learned.

"Hey *guy*, how's it going? Good to see you, *dude*! What's happenin' *wild man*?"

After escorting a patient to ER II *the long way* (for the third time), the triage nurse asked why I was not using the other door. I sheepishly admitted I did not have the code. She said it was the same for *both* doors...you just had to jiggle the handle upwards while punching the code on that particular door.

Silly me...how did I miss that?

Well, okay, I felt better now.

My first time through ER II, I walked briskly so no one would suspect I was on the verge of being lost. I decided if I came to a dead end, I could pretend I was going there on purpose, and then just turn around and keep walking.

Emerson was right, there really is safety in your speed.

I found myself standing in front of a linen supply cabinet with an unmarked and closed door on the far wall. I was trying to find my way out, but was it a closet?...the doctors' lounge?...a sterile nursery room?

A nurse glanced my way while washing her hands at a sink.

I decided I had gone too far to turn around now, so I strode confidently to the door and turned the handle...

...the hall...yea, I made it!

I sometimes helped transport patients to their rooms once the decision had been made to admit them.

One night we were pushing an 80's grandmother with a broken hip.

Once at the end of the longest hallway, we would make a left turn and then push hard to get the gurney up an incline. Right at the very top of the *hill*, a raised seam in the green, vinyl flooring always made the gurneys *jolt* while passing over.

It reminded me of a hasty, asphalt fill-in job after a city road crew had replaced a broken water main.

Our ancient and wounded passenger really felt the bump and cried out in pain.

I once read a book written by a Jewish, New York doctor titled, "Kill As Few Patients As Possible." I guess it was his way of following the old Socrates admonition to *do no harm.*

I figured this old gal had seen enough hard days in her lifetime that the hospital did not need to be adding to them.

I looked for, and found, a stack of forms on top of the microwave in the nurse's break room on which to report *broken equipment.*

I pulled a form from the middle of the stack, since the top half had round, coffee mug stains.

I was hoping they might work for the *floor,* as well as for a broken *ventilator.*

A couple of weeks later, I noticed workers installing all new flooring in the hallways, with *no seams.*

It was a lovely shade of light green, with dark green stripes and white specks. I am not sure how much my note had to do with it, but I decided to assume *full credit.*

That particular back hallway led to the volunteer check-in monitor where I would clock in at the beginning of each shift. In the future, every time I reached the top of that particular incline, I *stomped* on the floor where that seam used to exist.

This was *my* hallway.

My favorite nurse, ol' *Mud Face,* told me to check things out up on the *roof.*

She told me about an open-air, covered patio up there that was a cool place to take a break (and hide out). In the elevator, I noticed an "R" button, after the "9" for the ninth floor.

I gathered that meant *roof,* and not *return.*

When stepping out of the elevator, I found myself in a small room with doors all around, but no signs on the doors. I went for the largest door on the left, which opened into another small corridor, and more doors at the end.

I wasn't sure about this, but I trusted ol' *Mud Face* to not steer me wrong.

And sure enough, those doors led to this beautiful little oasis up there on top of the world.

It had the feel of being in a regular room, but with the wind blowing through once in a while. Clear, Plexiglas panels had been installed on the sides all around, offering a clear view to the freeway and beyond. A person could sit at one of the round tables while sipping on a Coke from the machine near the wall.

Two restrooms were also available. I could stay up here for a long time...until someone lit a cigarette.

Oh yeah, this was probably where all the smokers came to do their thing. I am sure the smokers knew how offensive their habit would be here at a *hospital*. They usually stayed off to one side and away from others.

I was amazed at the number of nurses who smoked. Why would a health-care professional do this to their body? I suspect to many nurses, this profession was just a *job* and had little to do with caring for sick people. I knew doctors who smoked as well...go figure.

The roof patio had space heaters overhead, but I could not find a switch. This was one of the areas where my mechanical knowledge came to my rescue.

I knew the Coke machine needed to be plugged into an electrical outlet, and a controller for the space heaters would also need the same *juice*. So, on a hunch, I looked *behind* the Coke machine... *voila*, there it was...the round knob with a pointer and a scale that registered from *zero* to *sixty*. They had it hidden pretty good.

At night, I was often the only person to venture to the roof for my fifteen-minute break at 10:00 PM. And it was often a bit chilly up there as I rested while working up enough nerve to finish my four-hour stint.

Once I knew how to turn the heaters on, I was as happy as a pig in slop.

As I learned the lay of the land in the ER, I noticed certain gurneys would sometimes be missing from their normal spots...usually hallway stations, V, VI and VII.

Miss Mud Face again was a great help as she explained how gurneys might often be left on the floors after a patient-transport.

So when returning from my break on the roof, I would take the stairs and poke my nose into each corridor as I made my way back down. Any errant gurneys would be rolled to an area near the elevators...where the stair doors opened.

This was another chore I could handle which no one else had the time to do. I was feeling more valuable all the time.

After a while, I only needed to stroll through the ER *manor* once, and I would immediately know if any of my *children* were missing. I was feeling better all the time as I discovered there were a few things I could do on my own.

The main hospital sat between two other buildings...one for pregnant mothers and infants...the other for children and kids to the age of sixteen. I had been told (*Mud Face* again) all three buildings were connected by tunnels.

I envisioned dark caves with a track and dirty coal carts, like in old mining movies.

So, one night, after I had all the gurneys tucked in for the night, I set out to find these *tunnels*.

I was instructed to go to the cafeteria, head downstairs, and start looking for signs on the walls that should lead me to the pregnant mothers. And sure enough, downstairs from the cafeteria, there were signs pointing the way.

To my disappointment, there were no railway tracks or coal carts...just a long corridor that ran outside the main building. I followed it as far as the information desk in the other building.

That wasn't so hard.

I then returned to the main building to search for the second *tunnel* to the children's building.

Miss M. Face said I should find it on the second floor behind Radiology where broken gurneys were often left. I wasn't sure I was there, but there was indeed a very long hallway where she indicated...with a couple of broken gurneys...but no signs to mark the way this time.

Again...no rails or coal carts. But I wasn't as surprised this time.

I began walking down another corridor until reaching an elevator. M. Face said I would need to take that elevator down one floor, and then she wasn't sure from there.

To make a long story short, I entered three conference rooms, two closets and one nursery (Ooops) before finding the children's ER. I wanted to locate that ER in case I ever needed to run an errand over there.

I thought I could re-trace my steps back to the long corridor through which I had come. I am convinced someone moved the building all around after I had passed through, because I never did find it.

I finally had to find a door that led to the street (not an easy task either) and returned using the sidewalk.

M. Face said she always had to do that as well, so I was not feeling too badly about it.

Often times, patients who came through the ER went straight

to Surgery or Intensive Care. And often times, a patient's chart needed to be rushed to ICU...a good job for *ER-Volunteer-Man*. So I was given the door code to that section as well.

I felt a bit funny my first time going in there.

I knew they had patients in there who were in bad shape...hence the word, *Intensive*. I was sent there by higher powers, so I punched in the code, walked in like I knew what I was doing and announced I was delivering a patient's chart.

For some reason, I was always expecting them to ask, "...and just *who* are you, and how did you get in here?" But that never happened...much to my surprise.

Occasionally, I was asked to return the *Intubation kit* to *Dirty Supply* to be repacked. That kit, and others had to be kept sterile at all times.

Clean and *Dirty* supply were located next to one another in the basement.

I was given the door codes for both areas, but warned to observe the markings on the floor and to never venture past them. I could do that.

For the longest time, I was taking the *long route* to get down there. *M. Face* again came to my assistance by showing me a shortcut down a back hallway the cafeteria-supply people used.

I felt like an old hand once I knew that route...through a set of double doors marked, "Official Personnel Only" (yes, that was *me*); down the hall...through an old exit door on the right with a well-worn brass doorknob...down the stairs...and then exiting into a hallway immediately in front of *Clean Supply*.

I was beginning to feel pretty smug about this.

I had *door-codes,* my own *hallway floor*, and I knew how to reach three buildings without getting into the rain (not counting re-

Joseph Apple

turning from children's ER).

ER PROPER

I was once asked what type people were seen in the ER? If you can "think it," that's the sort of patients I saw...everything from a *splinter* to a *scalping*.

The *scalping* happened when a drunk missed a turn in the country and drove his Ford Pinto through the woods, shearing the top from the car...as well as the top of his head.

When the paramedics called while enroute, they reported the top of the car to be missing...and that *they* didn't do it.

The old buzzard's scalp was lying on the gurney, still connected to the top of his head by a thin strip of tissue. I was curious as to how the surgeon was going to deal with this mess? The patient was talking to us and joking around. I doubted he was fully aware of his condition.

I also smelled alcohol.

The surgeon wanted to be sure all foreign material had been cleared from the wound underneath the still-attached portions of scalp, so he pulled out what looked like a *shower wand* and hooked it up to a sort-of garden hose.

He stuck the *shower wand* in one hole and began spraying.

Water and blood began flying everywhere, so I grabbed "splash gowns" and began dressing the nurses while they worked. The ER was really busy that night, so there was little time to prepare for this guy before he arrived.

When working closely together in the trauma room, all of us were often crawling over one another as we tended to the injured party.

This was no time to be embarrassed about making contact with the *Bobsy Twins* as the nurses and I jostled for position.

On another night, a man and woman were airlifted in from a remote hillside after a midnight horse ride had gone awry.

For some reason (we seldom knew the reasons) the horse had thrown both parties down a steep embankment. The male party had a moderate back injury, while the female had cuts and bruises... only *minor* injuries for her.

I love the term, *minor injuries.*

All that means is, most likely the injured party is not going to die from his or her injuries. My opinion is, a minor injury is an injury that happens to *someone else.*

The *real* problem soon surfaced when they begged us to not tell their *spouses.* Of course we had no control over that information.

They had made their beds and were now having to lie in them.

Midnight horseback rides are good ideas only in movies...and with your *own* spouse. Horses also appreciate a little light to see where they are going.

My job was to comfort the patients as much as possible. But what comfort can you give a guy with cracked vertebrae and looming divorce?

One night a Mexican field worker was airlifted in from an avocado ranch. I did not know how his injury happened, but his right, upper arm had been completely shredded.

The bicep muscles were open to the world, but with little blood to be seen.

The wound just did not look right.

Everything was a blackened, reddish color, like an old meaty T-bone left lying in the garbage the day after an expensive meal. I then learned the accident happened *three days ago.* For some reason, he was just now being seen for his injury.

Although Mexico is just across the border, the place is still a third-world country with marginal health care.

In the United States, emergency medicine still operates by the "golden hour" rule...meaning, if a patient can be seen within one hour of the incident, there is a good chance of survival.

I suspect Mexico operates on the principle of the "golden week."

I don't know why or how he was sent to us, but here he was.

I heard our ER surgeon consulting on the phone with a fellow surgeon, with the words *possible amputation* being tossed about. And as usual, once the patient had been rolled down the hallway, that would be the last I would see of him.

Someone else would be rolled in soon.

One thing I have learned about myself is that I am good when dealing with emergencies.

If I could jump from emergency to emergency and not have to deal with a leaky garage roof, or plugged toilet, I would be fine. Maybe that is why I enjoyed my Saturday nights in the ER? I don't know.

Meanwhile, someone else would be rolled in by fit young men and women dressed in dark blue uniforms who knew the ER door code by heart.

As a volunteer in the ER, I knew it was very important that I always inform the patients that I was NOT the doctor. And equally important, it was also vital that I not "touch" a patient in the wrong way.

I could lay my hand on a shoulder, or pat a back, but still had to be very careful even about that. But sometimes, a slight *touch* proved to be almost therapeutic.

One night a 13-yr-old female had been rushed in after her horse had fallen on top of her. The horse trail crossed an asphalt roadway at one point, and an automobile with loud exhaust spooked the animal. The horse reared up, and subsequently fell on top of the young girl.

She lay there, with cervical collar still in place, looking up at me with wide-open, frightened eyes. As I spoke with her, she told me of a previous injury while on her favorite horse which left her with a steel rod in her femur. She was afraid something had been re-injured. But her *real* fear was that her parents were going to make her stop riding her beloved horse.

As we waited for her to be taken to radiology for an *MRI* (expensive X-ray), I brushed some dirt from her cheek and placed my hand on her forehead for a few seconds. I uttered a soft prayer, asking God to intervene in her situation. She seemed very distraught and scared.

I had to leave her to care for others, but was surprised and delighted to see her much later that night *walking* out with her parents. The X-rays were all negative, with no fractures found.

She looked at me and asked if I was the one who had "touched" her. I confessed to having been the "toucher." She thanked me profusely as they walked out the door.

I wondered to myself if God might have actually healed her at my request? I don't know. It was clear to me that she, along with her parents thought I had done something special. I will never know.

I was just doing what my own mom would have done for me.

Talking to patients in the ER can be a risky job. Not *everyone* wants to chat while waiting to be stitched up...especially after being smacked on the head with a bottle of *Jack Daniels*.

And sometimes, the patients are scared out of their wits from sudden chest pains that could mean a complete change to their world as they know it.

But then again, some just want to talk.

I remember a 30's gal one night who was one of those who really did want to talk. She had a malady that had robbed her of the use of both legs. Her condition led to frequent visits to the ER and she seemed bored. She had neatly-styled blonde hair, a thin face, and spoke with a sexy, laid-back Southern drawl.

After my customary introduction, we hit it off as we discussed books, religion and medical stuff. But she was especially well-versed in religious matters, so we spent a lot of time talking about the Bible.

It was seldom that a patient wanted to actually talk about religion, and I did my best to hang in there.

After a while, she asked if I believed in *demons*?

I don't have any personal experience with demons, except possibly my third grade teacher, Mrs. *lardbutt* Magill...but I conceded they could exist.

She seemed to believe she was possessed by a demon of some sort...but did not elaborate on which type...*lardbutt*, or *fiery*?

She also asked me if I ever *prayed*, which I admitted to doing once in a while. And wouldn't you know it, she wanted *me* to pray for *her*. I had been advised by our volunteer director to steer clear of religion, but this gal seemed different.

Joseph Apple

So I agreed to pray for her. But she then asked if I could also *exorcise* her demon as well?

Well, that was a tall order.

I believe in God and all, but had never personally tried my hand at demon exorcism. For some strange reason, the authors of my volunteer manual steered clear of this subject, so I seemed to be on my own.

I decided to give it a shot, but no guarantee... hey, I'm just a volunteer here.

This was a hospital where people got help with their medical issues. I guessed this could be the right place to do this...but wasn't sure. But if she was serious about it, then I would do my best.

Jesus said it was peoples' *faith* in God that healed them, and she seemed to have it. So here goes...

I prayed a simple and quiet prayer for my Kentucky-sister's health issues, and tacked on as a side-request the thing about the demon.

Had I been more experienced at this, I suppose I could have smacked her on the forehead and yelled, "Be healed!" But I felt under-qualified for such a maneuver. I wanted to leave such moves to the *professionals*.

As with everyone else, she moved on after that night and I never saw her again. I often wish I knew how she fared with her demon?

I hope God was listening that night and nailed it for her.

People don't die in the emergency room as often as they do on TV.

If they are going to expire, they usually do it before arriving. Once there though, all effort is taken to make sure it does **not** happen inside the building. After all, when a patient passes on to the *great beyond* inside the ER, a lot of paperwork is generated that most doctors would rather avoid.

But once in a while, it was just going to happen no matter who is at the wheel of the ship.

I had just checked in at 8:00 p.m. as usual, but noticed odd behavior from nurse *big-arms* as she exited from behind the closed curtain of "bed six."

She peered back through the curtain for a moment and paused… but said nothing…and then resumed her normal activity.

One of my functions in the ER was to comfort patients and tend to their emotional needs, so I was allowed to enter on my own… which I did.

The "seventy's male" was lying motionless on the gurney with a breathing tube in place. His distraught adult daughter hovered over him like a honey bee over a dandelion, whispering things into his ear.

She sported a white, plastic photo ID tag clipped to the front of her cream-colored silk blouse, as though she had hurried here from behind a counter at a Hertz rent-a-car booth at the airport.

Her tears and reddened eyes spoke a language that no one in their right mind wants to hear. She was on her own, and very lost.

I had learned to tread very softly when in this type of situation. The normal reaction is to turn around and run as fast as you can. But this was my place, and I would do my best to comfort her as her dad coasted to a *stop.*

His shiny black shoes, black dress slacks, nylon over-the-calf socks and pin-striped shirt were in a plastic patient-belongings bag underneath the gurney.

He continued to sport a worn wedding band on his left hand as a stark reminder that earlier in the afternoon, he had been a part of the regular world, breathing the very same oxygen that every

Joseph Apple

other living person shared.

As she turned to me and asked what to expect next, I instinctively moved to her side and placed one arm around her shoulder. She leaned hard on me...a total stranger...and released a mournful cry.

The overhead monitor indicated heart activity, but it was clear no one was *home.*

I realized everything had been done that could be done, and now it was time to wait for the *bright light* at the end of the tunnel to make its appearance.

Of course, no one knows what the *bright light* really looks like up close. I doubt anyone wants *the big one* shining on them.

I shared with her, as I had been taught, that the sense of *hearing* was the very last to stop working when a person was dying and that he might still hear her.

So she whispered more things into his ear...as the heart monitor continued to beep.

She then pulled out her cell phone, called her sister and held the phone to his ear.

The blips on the monitor began hiccupping, with longer pauses between beats.

She turned to me once again and stood with me as we both stared at the monitor suspended above the bed on the wall...with longer spaces between the blips.

It was as though we were watching a truck that had crashed through a bridge guard rail and now teetering high above a river....rocking back and forth. I placed my arm around her once again and held her securely.

And then... the jagged green lines on the screen suddenly turned into one long, straight line with a steady tone...and no more blipping.

It was a sacred moment.

A life had just come to an end… and he was gone.

I thought she might fall apart then, but that did not happen.

Her worrying was now over.

A nurse stepped in, turned the monitor and ventilator off, and delivered instructions on what would take place next.

There was nothing more for me to do in that situation, so I returned to the hallway and began cleaning a gurney for another patient. It all seemed so surreal as a life suddenly ceased in front of my eyes.

On Monday morning I would be at work changing brake pads on a Ford van in a world far removed from this one. I would not be attending the funeral that was sure to follow, nor would I see this woman again with whom I had just shared a sacred moment.

All I could do was hope I had helped another human being through a dark moment.

But, ready or not, it was time to move on…the earth was still spinning.

After restocking linens and supplies in all the bedside cabinets, the ER doctor on duty came to me and asked if I could go to *bed two* and *work my magic* over there?

The ER doctors were always very busy and never spoke to me, and I doubted they even knew I existed. So I was very surprised the doctor was aware of my presence…and even more surprised to hear him suspecting me of possessing *magical powers* of some sort?

Nevertheless, I was impressed at such language. So I hurried to *bed two* to see what was needed. Upon drawing back the heavy gray curtain, there lay a mid-thirties female in great pain, screaming and trying to climb out of her bed.

I made eye-contact with her and asked what was wrong? She began yelling to me about harsh treatment from all the other staff and that no one cared about her.

I asked about her problems, and listened as she described her abdominal pains that would come-and-go. I asked if she was cold... and offered to get her a warm blanket. At first, she refused...then said *maybe* she could use a blanket.

I hurried and fetched a warm blanket from the blanket warmer. She had stopped yelling and trying to climb out of her bed, so that was a little progress.

I spread the warm blanket over her and playfully tucked it under her chin, sharing about how my own mom used to do that to me when I was a kid.

It is hard to tuck a blanket under your own chin without getting your own arms outside of the blanket and getting cold again.

I smoothed her dirty, blonde hair out of her eyes and asked if she wanted a tissue to blow her nose? After she had blown her nose, I pressed the warm blanket even more securely under her chin while asking if she had any kids?

She said her daughter was home watching the dog. I asked about the dog, and she said it was a golden retriever who would steal plastic flowers from their neighbor's porch and bring to her house.

I then listened as she talked about her no-good husband, his parents and her previous divorce. She seemed to have a ton of problems which I was powerless to solve....me, the mechanic with the C in biology.

I glanced up and caught a glimpse of the ER doctor around the edge of the curtain... smiling.

I had no idea what I was doing, but she was no longer screaming and crying.

I didn't feel like anything *magical* was happening, but she had at least calmed down.

Her nurse then returned and took her to radiology for X-rays, so my job was done. If there was any magic in what I had done, I was certainly not seeing it. I had just listened and tried to make her feel better.

But then I got to thinking...maybe I had something after all that no one else had?

I continued with my work and replaced three empty containers of sanitary wipes in ER 4.

On my way back, another nurse stopped me in the hallway and asked my help with a *screamer* in the private room? I was feeling pretty good about myself by then and jumped to *work my magic* on yet another patient.

There she was...an old gray-haired gal who looked to be about 75-years-old.

I moved in close so she could see my smiling face.

I inquired about her problems and listened as she complained.

I agreed with everything she said and tried to work in a story about my kids and our own dog, Corky...a husky, and how we would have to chase him all over the beach to get him back home.

She had stopped screaming, and was staring intently into my face.

She then held up one hand as though motioning for me to move in closer.

Frightened patients sometimes found it comforting to touch my face.
So I moved in close...

...as she then SLAPPED me across the cheek and said she did not care about me, my kids OR my dog and wanted to go home!

...so much for my *magical powers.*

Needless to say, that brought me back down to earth pretty fast. Just then, her nurse returned with a family member who would stay with the old battle-ax.

No one had seen what had taken place, and for all her nurse knew, I had indeed worked my *magical powers*, since the old gal had clammed up.

So I quickly and rudely learned about the hazards of believing in my own *magic.*

Even Houdini sometimes ran into trouble after becoming over-confident and pushing the envelope, so I felt I wasn't alone.

I figured it might be best if I paid no attention to what the others said and just did what I knew to do...

...whatever that was?

THE TRAUMA ROOM

A h, the trauma room.

This was where all the really cool stuff took place. Everyone wanted to be in the trauma room.

But I was scared of the trauma room and not sure if I was allowed inside.

Mud Face again to the rescue.

She slipped up behind me as I peeked through the crack between the heavy, windowless doors, and encourage me to go on in.

The room contained two gurneys anchored to special securements on the floor. Each gurney also had a special tray that would hold x-ray film to gather images of broken legs and spines. Overhead was a rail fastened to the ceiling on which a radiographic scanner could be quickly maneuvered to any position desired.

Between the gurneys stood two leaded glass panels on wheels. The glass panels would deflect stray X-ray beams, providing a protective barrier for observers after a head-on smash between the semi-trailer and Ford Escort.

The room was fully stocked to handle everything from open-heart surgery to a point-blank, twelve-gauge shotgun blast.

This was where I wanted to spend my time...in the *trauma room*.

M. Face pushed me on in and told me to stay behind the glass panels.

I had been invited... I had permission to be here.

I watched closely as the surgeon and trauma team worked together. Everyone had a task to perform. This was trauma team, *Alpha*. Trauma team *Bravo* worked in rotation with team *Alpha*.

I felt as though I had just been invited into a secret chamber of horrors where forbidden acts were to take place...acts never viewed by the general public... and I had just been ushered in.

One nurse monitored an IV as isotonic saline fluid coursed through a number 12 needle, into the median cubital vein of the forearm. Another nurse watched closely as oxygen was being forced through a hose into the freshly-intubated trachea, inflating the patient's lungs.

A lab tech was drawing blood to be rushed to the lab upstairs for rapid evaluation. The surgeon was carefully inserting a wire into the patient's chest and into the pulmonary vein over which a tube would be inserted to allow an even faster influx of fluids.

Two x-ray technicians flittered over the patient like butterflies gathering nectar, sliding films underneath broken limbs to gather images as quickly as possible. Everyone had a job to perform as the surgeon calmly gave directions.

This was the *golden hour* where the patient's life teetered on the fence between life and death. I watched the trauma surgeon's face as he gathered all the data and gave instructions to the nurses. He looked every bit like a general directing the troops into battle.

I was captivated by all that I was observing.

But when the surgeon withdrew the small guide wire from the patient's chest, I felt my face flush...or rather, *un-flush* as most of the blood in my body began settling around my ankles.

At that time, I did not know exactly what he was doing and it was all beginning to get to me.

I recalled when I was a child and hanging around the garage at night while my dad worked.

Our small community of Oaklandon, Indiana had one auto shop in the center...next to the barber shop... across the street from the drug store and Legion Hall with the fire station on the other corner.

The swinging boom on the tow truck had smacked my dad in the head, resulting in a neat, v-shaped gash on the top of his head. It bled a lot as he pressed a clean shop towel down hard to curb the flow.

He grabbed a phone receiver with the other hand and called Dr. Miller at home. The doctor's office was just behind the garage and we would walk over as soon as we saw the headlights of Dr. Miller's Pontiac bounce as he crossed the railroad tracks.

We followed Dr. Miller into the building as he unlocked the doors and flipped on the lights.

I was soon watching as he sat my dad down and cleaned his wound. I saw the blood running through my dad's hair and down the back of his neck. Dr. Miller was laughing and joking with Dad the whole time as he asked about a vibration he was getting in the front of his car.

I was starting to feel a little hot.

Dr. Miller pulled out a small vial of Lidocaine, inserted a syringe and withdrew the deadening fluid. He squirted some of the liquid out, gave it a tap with the index finger on his left hand, and then began jabbing directly into the gaping wound on my Dad's head.

This was my first time to watch such a procedure, and I was taken aback by the way I was starting to feel. I then began to notice the smells of the office and how strong they had suddenly become.

As soon as he had jabbed the pain killer into my Dad's scalp, he grabbed a curved needle with black thread and began sewing the wound closed...poking the needle directly into the bleeding flesh.

I noticed how my Dad flinched with the first couple of stitches... and then my head began to feel like when I was stuck on the merry-to-round at our school's playground with one of the big kids making it go around as fast as he could make it go.

I realized I needed to get off this thing, and I needed to get off NOW.

But I wanted to be a *man* about this and not let anyone know I was in trouble. I noticed how Dr. Miller looked over at me... and then asked if I wanted to step outside into the cool air?

I didn't need to be asked that question twice...as I turned and headed for the door. I was always puzzled at how he knew I was in trouble? Of course, I now know I must have looked like *Casper the Ghost* after all the blood had left my face.

When the trauma surgeon withdrew the guide wire from the patient's chest, I felt my *merry-to-round* starting to speed up. I knew it was time to get off.

I glanced at my watch and pretended I needed to be somewhere else...*anywhere else.*

I shuffled down the hallway to the supply room and sat on a cardboard case of toilet paper rolls until my blood found its way back to all its usual places.

I had not had this happen in a long time and was a bit disturbed by it all. I really wanted to work in this setting, but was not going to be of much help when spending half my time sitting on a box of toilet paper in the supply closet.

I decided to jump right back on the *horse* and return to the *arena*. But this time, I decided to not look at certain parts of what they were doing.

I wasn't ready for it just yet.

The radio room was right next to the trauma room where we could listen in and hear what was on the way.

I overheard the words, *multiple gunshot wounds,* which always got everyone excited.

I am sure the staff got into this business to help people, but after seeing it day after day, they got used to it and looked forward to something interesting once in a while.

I soon heard the *monotone* words of an operator's voice coming from the speakers in ceilings all over the hospital...

"Trauma team Alpha...report to the Emergency Department..."

She would always repeat that command two more times. The members of team Alpha began showing up and slipping on leaded vests.

The trauma surgeon was soon there as well. Everyone stood around and waited for the paramedics to wheel the victim inside.

... the *calm* before the storm.

I made myself useful by holding the doors open. As soon as the shooting victim was rolled in, the *blood guys* began inserting large-bore IVs into the African-American male's arms.

The lead paramedic then began reciting the story of what they had found at the scene and everything they had done to the patient so far. As the surgeon removed the blood-stained white sheet covering the victim, I noticed small dots all over the victim's body where blood was seeping out.

He had places on his arms, legs, shoulder, one foot, and one hand.

I was asked to grab some towels from a cabinet... and then to throw mats on the floor to soak up some of the blood. The physician-assistant on staff was called in to assist. Everyone was crawling over one another to save this guy's life.

Someone said his wounds looked as if he was running away from something as another person used him for target practice with a 9mm pistol.

Had a drug deal just gone bad? Was this guy an innocent by-stander to someone else's problem? Did his girlfriend do this?

I learned that the health workers in the ER seldom knew the answers to these questions.

I then realized that once I had been included in working on the victim, all the blood did not bother me.

I could look at the holes in his legs without my *merry-go-round* even beginning to move. I was then directed to help position the patient's arms for x-rays. The surgeon suggested that I grab a lead vest from a hook on the wall.

...ME...the volunteer.

I was being included as part of the team. I followed the radiologist's directions so he could get the exact picture of the limbs he was after.

This guy was in bad shape, but he was still very lucky. The bullets had missed all of his vital organs. As soon as his vital signs were stable, the surgeon began counting all the bullet holes.

I looked hard myself to see if I could visualize what had happened.

He had a hole through the palm of one hand... as though he had thrown one hand up to protect himself from the shooter. He also had a bullet entry point in his left shoulder...maybe the same bullet that had passed through his hand?

He had a hole on the outside of his left thigh...and I could see another hole on the inside of that same thigh.

And then I could see how the skin of his scrotum was partly torn, with yet another hole in the other thigh.

As the surgeon rubbed his thumb over the torn skin of the scrotum... I winced, thinking of how close this guy had come to losing the *family jewels!* It had only been a glancing blow to the private parts. The bullet was lodged in the right thigh where it caused more carnage.

The surgeon decided to count all the holes to make sure they had not missed anything. He took what looked like a large Q-tip and began exploring all the holes and noting their direction.

He counted eight holes.

I thought sure he had missed the one at the guy's right ankle and held out my gloved index finger to politely point it out...and he said to his PA, "nine."

I felt good about that. I realized that even though I was not one of the trained professionals, I still had a brain in my head and could pay attention to what was in front of us.

This guy would need surgery, and it was the immediate job of the trauma staff to get the guy stabilized and do all that could be done right there. He was about ready to go, so I was given another order to run down the hall and get the elevator open and locked in place.

The operating rooms or, OR, were upstairs, and things needed to happen quickly. I ran to do that job, and was feeling more important all the time.... me, the volunteer/automobile mechanic.

They had plenty of people to take the patient on from there, so my part was finished... as small as it was. I returned to help clean up the mess, but felt proud that I had just helped to save a life.

...never mind that he might have been a drug dealer, thief, or killer... I had just helped to save a life, and that felt good.

But I was new to this world, and it would be a while before I would come to grips with the senseless carnage people could inflict on one another.

AN AQUAINTANCE

I thought I recognized the guy I passed in the hallway as the triage nurse escorted him and his son into the ER.

He looked at me twice as well, as though we might have met at a garage sale or something. I followed them to the gurney where his son sat on the edge of the bed.

The young boy, about nine years of age, had a cloth wrapped around one hand with a black string sticking out. As the nurse removed the cloth, I then saw the problem...a fish hook! The *string* was fishing line that had been cut from the reel.

The nurse began cleaning the hand with hydrogen peroxide and sterile saline solution as his dad and I watched. His dad then looked harder at me and said,

"Don't I know you from somewhere?"

I admitted that he looked very familiar as well.

After trading occupations, it then hit us both...he worked behind the counter at a local auto parts store where I had purchased parts in my own work for my employer.

We had indeed worked together. He seemed to relax a bit once he knew he had a *friend* in the ER.

I explained to him why I was there and what I was trying to do. I

Joseph Apple

am sure it felt good to him to run into a friend in a place as foreign as the emergency room of a hospital.

This would happen several more times in the ER as I spent my Saturday nights here over the course of the next eleven years. I realized everyone could use a *friend* when in the emergency room. And that's what I was trying to do with patients...be a friend.

The dad and I joked about our jobs and talked about other guys we knew in the auto business. We both agreed that people were really getting the shaft when taking their cars to the local *Lube and Screw* for a smog test.

The son still had the fish hook imbedded in his finger, but he was taking it pretty well so far.

Before long, the doctor on duty took a look, and knew exactly what needed to be done. After a thorough cleaning, he injected with good old Lidocaine to deaden the finger before pushing the hook on through and cutting the barbed end off with a pair of wire cutters. It was then a simple matter of backing the hook out...*without* the barbed end and applying a sterile dressing.

The son certainly did not like the needle with pain deadener...or the tetanus shot. But once those parts were over, the rest was a piece of cake. They were both very happy after the hook had been removed.

Fish hooks in *skin* is a VERY big deal when it is your own, or your son's skin we are talking about.

I saw them out the door, and a good time was had by all...except for possibly the son.

It struck me that THIS was why I was here. I was able to help take the sting out of someone else's *hard time*.

DOCTOR JOHN

I seldom saw the same ER workers on back-to-back Saturday nights.

They seemed to work in shifts that ran their cycle every three weeks. It took a while to get to know everyone. Even then, I did not know anyone very well.

I was only here for four hours on Saturday nights.

John, the tall male nurse who supervised the trauma room seemed to take a liking to me.

He was older than most of the other nurses and had a definite *doctor* persona about him. He seemed to enjoy having me around as his *personal assistant.* He would often direct me to gather the vital signs on one of his patients, which I loved to do.

I wanted to be used and to learn all I could, so this was the perfect arrangement.

I had taken the necessary emergency medical training and had achieved my California EMT certificate. I had not actually used my EMT training in a place of employment, but at some point in my future, I really wanted to work in the area of emergency medicine.

I already had a good job and career as an automobile mechanic, so I was not about to change careers and work for *less* money. Besides, EMTs were mostly used to transport old geezers from nursing homes to their doctor's appointments.

I was a *volunteer*, but since I had the training and California certification, John used me when he was working triage. He often had me gather the patient's vitals as he typed information into the computer... blood pressure, temperature, heart rate, blood oxygen saturation levels and respiration rates.

I was **really** doing this... working in the trenches and using *live ammunition*.

At John's direction, I had just called in a middle-aged female from the waiting room.

...ME...the automobile mechanic...had just opened the door to the waiting room and called out a patient's name to come forward.

The guys back at the shop would be blown away to see what I was doing just now. This wasn't checking tire inflation on the plumber's van...this was the real deal.

I had her sit as I wrapped the blood pressure cuff around her right bicep. We used an automated BP machine in gathering the measurements for the sake of standardization.

I placed a protective sheath on the oral temperature probe and placed under her tongue and pushed some buttons. At the same time, I clipped a probe over her index finger to measure her blood oxygen saturation levels.

John was typing rapidly while asking questions of the red-faced woman. I was so busy gathering her base physical information that I wasn't paying a lot of attention as to why she had even come here in the first place.

When the blood pressure gauge registered a pressure of 220/180, my eyes bugged out. I had never seen a blood pressure that high.

John, still focusing on the keyboard, softly mentioned that unless I said something, he would assume everything was okay with the vitals.

WHOA... I suddenly felt a bit of responsibility. This was no game.

I recognized this to be a life-and-death situation, and my actions could have a direct impact on the patient's life. The recommended blood pressure for an adult has always been 120/80, and recently lowered to 115/75.

So *220/180* meant the air hose had been left clipped to the valve stem too long and this whole thing could blow at any second.

As a heart pumps blood through arteries, it is very much like pumping air into a bicycle tire with a tire pump. Each stroke of the pump is like that top number of "115" when the pump is activated. The bottom number of "75" would be the pressure already in the tire, or arteries. The top number reflects *systole*, meaning, contraction. The bottom number reflects *diastole,* or, dilation... when the heart chambers refill.

I knew all these things from my training. But to actually see someone sitting beside me with pressure readings like this was a whole new ballgame.

Had she been a truck tire, I would have run!

Her smallest arteries, usually in the brain, could let go at any time causing a stroke...or *worse.*

I wasted no time and quickly alerted John to what I was seeing.

He just as quickly led her to a gurney and had her lie down.

He stopped everything else he was doing to grab the ER physician on duty to get meds into this gal to keep her from *blowing.*

That was a real eye-opener for me.

So far, I was just a volunteer around here and had no real responsibilities. But if I was going to be used *for real*, I figured hey, I better get with the program.

So, from then on, I *eyeballed* every person real hard as soon as I laid eyes on them. I mean, I knew the basic things to look for. And it wasn't like I was doing it on my own authority... I mean, I was always working under someone else.

But from that point on, I never assumed a person was okay just because they were *walking* and *talking*.

John had me call the next patient.

He was an old dude, brought in by his adult son.

The son seemed to be about my age... maybe a couple of years younger. The old guy looked to be about my own dad's age... gray hair, scruffy jeans, red flannel shirt... somewhere in his seventies. The old dude was cradling his left arm with his right hand and said his arm hurt.

The son explained that he thought his dad needed to get more exercise and had bought him a bicycle. I thought to myself...

"A bike? He's an old man... what are you trying to do.... kill him?"

I mean, I ride a bike in my triathlon events, and it is not a simple thing to jump back on a bike after not having ridden one in many years. You're going to dump it a couple of times and fall into the bushes once in a while.

I figured the son was not the sharpest *knife* in the drawer.

After gathering the old dude's vitals... gathering his blood pressure from the *other* arm...I helped him into a wheelchair and pushed him around the corner to radiology. They would take X-rays to see what the arm looked like.

The old guy didn't seem to be in much pain, so I was suspecting a sprain of some sort. He had tenderness and some swelling of the upper arm, or humerus, but it did not seem to be too bad. I checked his radial pulse at the wrist of that same arm…which felt strong, so I determined the circulation to not be compromised. Nurse John agreed.

When they brought the X-ray around, I was shocked to see that his humeral shaft was completely broken off and displaced. I would never have guessed it was that bad by observing the old guy's re-actions. He just sat there and hardly said anything.

Had that been me, I would have been crying, screaming and climbing the walls.

But this old dude was just very quiet about it all.

That was another learning experience for me. Everyone reacts to pain differently, and not the same way I might react.

I remember when my own dad would skin a knuckle after a wrench accidentally slipped. He might say:

"Well, that *stung* a little."

And of course, that meant it hurt like crazy! Or if he said he *felt it*, or admitted to any sensation of pain at all, it could have been any-thing from a smashed finger to an amputated leg.

The old dude would require surgery to put the bone back to-gether, so they put the arm in a sling and made plans to admit him.

Oh, and the son?

I was right.

After talking to him more…he was an idiot.

MY PATIENTS

Once in a great while...maybe two or three times in eleven years, I was given a patient of my very own to oversee.

I am sure the volunteer coordinator would have cringed had she ever heard about this, but sometimes it would just happen.

A homeless gal had been brought in after being found in the bushes. She had been given a quick examination by the triage nurse and placed on a gurney in the hallway... ER VII.

This gal was asleep when I first saw her, with straw in her brown hair and dirt all over her thin brown jacket. She was wearing a man's blue-and-white, checked, long sleeved shirt with frayed material around the collar.

Her dark blue polyester, bell-bottom pants reminded me of a pair I once owned when I was in the mainstream of high fashion...*once upon a time.*

She reeked of alcohol and seemed to be asleep. Her nurse pulled me aside and asked if I could keep watch over "Nancy." Evidently, *Nancy* had been drinking, fell and hit her head on a rock, and then rolled down a hill. Someone had found her in the bushes.

There was probably more to the story than that...we very seldom learned the *whole* truth in any situation.

This was all we had to work with on her.

Nancy's nurse was also a member of trauma team Alpha, and another *trauma* was on its way just then. Since *Nancy* was drunk out of her skull *and* with a lump on the back of her head, her nurse needed to be sure she was remaining *with us* and not slipping into an irreversible coma.

So my job, should I decide to accept it, was to make sure Nancy could still be aroused once in a while. I felt I was up to the challenge.

I figured I better begin with a base-line reading, so I jostled her shoulder to arouse her.

"Hey Nancy!" I shouted into her ear.

"Can you tell me your name?"

"Waaa?", she mumbled.

"Can you tell me your name?" I shouted again.

"Naaanncccc," she slurred.

That was close enough. I decided her response was appropriate.

Normally, I would ask for *person, place and time.*

Did they know their name? Did they know where they were? And did they have any idea of the time or date? But since my job was to just make sure she was not slipping into a coma, I decided to go just with the name.

I went on about my regular duties of restocking the bedside cabinets and changing sheets on gurneys. But every fifteen minutes, I stopped to give Nancy another *shake...*

"Hey Nancy!...you still with us?"

"Huuuhhhh?"

Joseph Apple

"Okay, go back to sleep!"

It wasn't much, but still, I had my very own live patient to oversee. Maybe all volunteers started like this?

My second patient was assigned to me in the trauma room.

A drunk driver had run a red light and T-boned an old couple innocently driving through an intersection. As often happened, the drunk was not seriously hurt, while the elderly couple was really broken up and in critical condition.

Both the drunk abuser and the innocent female passenger from the other car were transported to us. Her husband was taken to another hospital. It just happened that way.

The *drunk* arrived first.

I overheard John, the trauma supervisor, apprising the surgeon of the situation.

All medical personnel are supposed to treat each patient equally, but when it comes to drunk drivers, I sensed it was hard to keep the emotions in check. I observed as the surgeon gave the *drunk* the customary head-to-toe evaluation.

He grabbed the *drunk's* neck and asked if he felt any pain back there?…and then on to each arm, leg and torso, as though searching for contraband in an inmate's cell mattress.

Once the trauma surgeon had *cleared* the *drunk* of serious injury, he was moved aside to make room for the elderly gal who was on her way. I then heard John discussing with the trauma surgeon the problem they were faced with.

They did not have enough trauma team members present to handle both patients under standard trauma protocol.

Once their huddle was over, John then came to me and said the drunk was *all mine!*

Wow, I was excited about that...my VERY own patient!

Never mind that he was the scourge of all society with not a single redeeming attribute to his name. He was now MY patient!....me, the automobile mechanic who would be replacing a muffler on a Ford Fairmont the next Monday at work.

The poor elderly gal was then rushed in by paramedics and everyone devoted their full attention to her ruptured spleen and broken pelvis...among other broken parts.

As for me, I had observed how quickly the trauma surgeon had checked off on the drunk and knew he could have missed a couple of things....like a missing *foot,* or *hand*? So I watched him carefully to see if he had any more serious injuries that might manifest themselves.

I shone a light into each pupil to look for equal and reactive pupil responses. They were slow to respond, but equal. I did some more feeling around on his limbs to make sure he had no hidden broken bones. He seemed to be *all there*, as the trauma surgeon had ascertained.

He had cuts on his face and arms, so I opened a bottle of sterile saline solution and hydrogen peroxide and began cleaning him up. I was fine when it came to cleaning up messes. So I was careful with him as I cleaned and asked if certain parts hurt?

I will always remember how he looked up at me with his wide-open eyes and remarked how I was the only person who was being been nice to him.

He didn't deserve the treatment I was giving him, nor did he know he had just been handed off to the *volunteer.* As far as the trauma staff was concerned, he didn't even deserve the bed space he was occupying.

I realized that this miserable wretch must have been an innocent little baby at some point, and maybe even had a mom as well? Although...I guess he *could* have been raised by wolves? It was clear he had made some really horrible choices that were an affront to all civilized people everywhere.

But he was *my* patient, and I was going to take care of him.

I whispered into his ear that things didn't have to be like this and that he could make a change for the better. He gripped my arm and said he would never forget me. But then again, he had been drinking and would probably not remember any of this tomorrow.

I was just doing what I thought was the right thing to do. I would like to believe there is hope for everyone.

The police were there, and I am sure this guy went straight to the slammer after being released from us.

And as with most of the other patients, I would never see this guy again.

DEATH TRANSPORT

I often helped with transporting patients to their rooms when being admitted.

The nurses were happy to have me, a guy with strong arms and back, to help move a patient.

I enjoyed doing something different as well. It did not require a lot of skill...just rolling them to the other end of the hospital, taking the elevator to the seventh, eighth or ninth floor, checking in at the nurse's station and then helping transfer the patient into a regular hospital bed.

I often did the job by myself once I had the routine down. Rules were in force as to who I could transport.

Anyone who was on a **monitor** was off limits to me, or any other volunteer.

Being on a heart monitor meant the patient was at risk for having a heart attack, or worse. This could very easily happen on a gurney during transport, requiring immediate medical attention.

Sometimes it would happen that the ER was so busy they could not spare anyone to transport a patient. They actually employed EMTs to do only that one thing...transport.

On Saturday nights, things could really get crazy.

I must admit, as tempting as it must have been, I don't recall anyone ever breaking that rule. However, one night it got *bent* a little.

They had a guy on a monitor ready to be taken to a room, but no one to transport. John then stepped in and suggested they let *me* take him.

They huddled in a corner of the room that night like football coaches contemplating sending in the third-string quarterback during a 40-0 *blowout.*

Surprisingly to me, they told me to go ahead and take him. I was very surprised that they were directing me to do this.

So I began moving him along, with heart monitor beeping steadily. Once I was away from everyone else and waiting for the elevator, I picked up his chart and glanced through it.

The words *palliative care* caught my eye.

I knew the word *palliative*...it meant he was there to *croak!*

If at any time the *big light* was seen at the end of the tunnel, we were supposed to step back and let it shine.

I guess they thought it would make little difference who was moving the old buzzard around when he went, so we might as well let the *volunteer* take him.

Let's not waste any of the paid help on this. But I didn't mind. I was learning something new all the time.

SAD STUFF

Sometimes I saw some truly sad sights in the ER.

I always tried to go from bed-to-bed to speak with the patients who wanted to talk. One night I stopped in at bed number seven and introduced myself as usual to a young man with Down Syndrome.

Down Syndrome, or *trisomy 21*, is a genetic defect where the fetus has an extra chromosome at position 21. People with this genetic defect have an assortment of mental and physical problems, including a degree of mental retardation.

I recognized the defect right away from the characteristic appearance of his face and the roundish features. This young man greeted me cheerfully:

"Hi, my name is Larry…what's your name?"

(me) "Well, my name is Joe. How are you?"

"My guts are coming out. Wanta see?"

At this, he drew back his top cover sheet, exposing reddish-brown intestines that were spilling out of his anus. They were in a large pile on a green pad as though he had just given birth to a space alien.

And no, I did NOT want to see.

Joseph Apple

He also told me he lived in a group home with several other mentally challenged kids. He didn't actually SAY he lived with several
others who were mentally challenged, but I could figure that out
on my own.

I was familiar with group homes for the disabled. I also was aware
of some of the problems encountered in homes that were not up
to state standards.

I learned later, as I had initially suspected, this poor kid had been
sexually abused in some fashion. His colon had been perforated
by an *object*, thus allowing his intestines to escape from his abdomen. I doubt he had the mental capacity to grasp the magnitude
of his situation...and it was probably just as well. Whoever did
this was a real sicko.

I had him pull the sheet back over his intestines as we carried on a
sort-of normal conversation about his friends in the home.

There was not much help I could provide in this situation, so I
excused myself and moved on. He was in the hands of the ER doctor, social workers and police, I assumed. The police were *always*
there on a Saturday night.

On another night, I could hear screaming in the waiting room as a
young unwed mother rushed in, carrying an infant in her arms.

The triage nurse quickly ushered her in to evaluate the problem.
The nurse took one look, then carried the baby into the trauma
room to lay on a gurney. I stepped in to watch and be ready in case
I was needed to rush to the pharmacy for medications at the far
end of the hospital.

The child looked to be about six months old and was unconscious, but still breathing. The poor thing lay motionless on
the gurney with both arms held rigidly above its head as though
being robbed at gunpoint. From my training, I recognized it right
away.

The baby was *posturing.*

When a child is suffering from a brain injury, the body sometimes responds by extending both arms overhead when the injury is affecting the whole brain or spinal cord. Sometimes the result is a *half posture* if only one side is affected.

This child was in *full-posture*, and that was not good at all.

The young mother said she had *dropped* the baby.

Our emergency department was not equipped to handle infants, so a specialist was called over from the children's hospital next door.

Maybe the young mother really had dropped her child? But, most likely, the baby had been shaken out of frustration, by herself, or a male friend to stop the crying. It happens often enough that it has a name...

...*The Shaken Baby Syndrome.*

The young mother was sobbing and shaking badly herself while watching a child that would not wake up.

My initial reaction was to think what a slob this mom was. Or, how could she let her boyfriend do such a thing?

I then remembered how tough it could be to satisfy a young child when the crying just won't stop. I also remembered the frustration of needing sleep myself when up in the middle of the night with our own son or daughter.

If I am honest with myself, I have to ask if this could possibly be *me* under the same circumstances?

But it wasn't.

And I don't want to think about it any longer.

I was glad I was just a volunteer and could move on to the next patient and try to forget about this one.

It was getting close to midnight and I could go home soon.

BAD THINGS HAPPENING TO GOOD PEOPLE

When first coming on duty, I would always peek into the trauma room to see if anyone was in there that night.

One night a mid-sixties guy lay on the gurney as the staff did their thing on him. I was always interested to learn what was wrong with each patient and what had brought them to the ER.

I observed as the surgeon began lightly pricking his lower extremities with a pin, asking if he felt anything?

I thought...oh, oh...this does not look good.

If the doctor has to *ask* if you are feeling something, that is never good.

One of the staff then told me how this guy was hanging Christmas lights on the outside of his house when his ladder slid sideways, causing him to fall twenty feet to the ground. He wasn't feeling anything below his waist.

No doubt he had a wife and kids, and probably grandkids as well who would be looking forward to a nice Christmas season. He was outside hanging the lights to get into the holiday spirit.

And then...WHAM.

It often happened suddenly and without warning. His life was forever altered in two seconds.

I looked into the waiting room to see if he had family out there. I did not see anyone who fit the description of what I thought his wife might look like. While running a pair of shoes to a recently admitted patient on the ninth floor, I passed a mournful group of people in the darkened main lobby.

The main lobby was closed at this time of the evening, so it was unusual to see family out there. Everyone was gathered around a *sixties* woman, dressed in a gray flannel coat. She was a little plump, and looked like she baked lots of pies....like "Aunt Bee" from the Mayberry TV show...you know, Sherriff Taylor's mom.

She was crying and holding a white hanky to her eyes. I walked past them, and then stopped in my tracks. I looked back and decided to interject myself and check on them.

Checking on people like this was always awkward for me. If I was wrong and did not know about their loved one, I would be stuck with them and powerless to do much. But I stuck my neck out and gave it a shot.

I gave my usual introductory spiel and asked about their situation. Sure enough, she was with the gentleman with the damaged spinal cord in the trauma room. I then shared with her how I had just been in the trauma room with her husband. I told her how he was talking to the surgeon and responding well to his questions.

I knew better than to say any more than that. The patient's medical condition and prognosis was for the surgeon to share. However, she already knew her husband could not move his legs after falling and suspected the worst. It was always very comforting to family when I could at least give them *some* information on their loved one.

The old gal often mentioned God, so I decided to stick my neck out a little further and offered to pray for her husband. I wasn't sure what I would say, but just felt it was the right thing to do just then.

I always hated to pray out loud when called upon in Sunday school. Praying was a private matter to me, plus I didn't want to sound stupid in front of other people.

My neck was already out there too far, so here goes....

I prayed a soft prayer for her husband, head bowed and with a hand on her shoulder. I don't remember what I said, but it seemed to do some good. She seemed to need a lot of comfort, and I tried to provide it.

I could only guess as to how their story ended, but I doubt it was very good. He probably spent the remainder of his life in a wheelchair in a nursing home. And she probably had to rely on the support of her adult children from that point on.

I thought it was a shame their Christmas had to be like this...just a shame.

SCREAMS IN THE NIGHT

I t was a slow night and everything seemed to be under control.

As I looked for something to do, I decided to take a walk and search for any misplaced gurneys. I took the elevator to the ninth floor, as I often did and began my search from there.

As soon as I had stepped from the elevator, I heard this loud and mournful *wailing* coming from somewhere on the floor. Some woman was screaming at the top of her lungs.

Once you hear this type of scream, you don't forget it.

It was not a short, loud scream like what you would hear from someone being frightened by a mean pit bull. Nor did it sound like a scream from someone falling off their back porch.

I have only heard this sort of scream when another human being was in the throes of death.

It was a bit unusual to hear screaming late at night on any of the floors. At 11:00 p.m., things were usually in order for the night. This was not the emergency room where I worked, so I did not pay that much attention to it.

Just then, the hospital's paid patient coordinator stepped around the corner. I had seen her in the ER a few times, but we had never spoken.

She always looked neat and professional in her dark blue skirt with matching jacket and white blouse. Her neatly styled blonde hair was always in order as though she had just sprayed it with an industrial-strength lacquer. The green cord around her neck which carried her hospital photo ID was the only thing that always looked out of place.

It was late and she looked tired.

I was surprised when she walked straight up to me and began talking like we were lifetime chums. She got right to the point and asked if I could somehow quiet the *screamer* and get her off the floor?

Yikes! That was a scary one for me.

I was very impressed she was asking my help...me, the automobile mechanic/volunteer with the C+ in Sociology. But still.... this was a tall request. I didn't want to disappoint her, so I agreed to give it a shot.

She led me to the room, and then disappeared. I suspected she had had a long day. I had no idea what I was going to do and was feeling very frightened just then. I walked on in and tried to get a bearing on the situation.

I had seen this type of patient in the ER several times...minus all the screaming.

The 80's, white-haired patient was laying there with her mouth wide open, eyes closed and gasping for air. It was evident the *shop* was out of business and no one was expected to return...most likely a stroke victim.

All the *noise* was coming from the adult daughter, with her husband standing helplessly by her side.

Who was I to step into this sort of situation? I had no idea what I was going to do.

I told *stiff hair* I would do something, so I needed to do *something*.

I took a deep breath and moved in close by her side. This felt odd to me, but I placed one arm around her shoulder and held her firmly. I mean, her husband was standing right there on the other side, so this felt creepy to me.

It was as though we were in a *cloud*, or some sort of time-warp where all the normal rules did not apply.

Her husband did not say, "Hey, what are you doing with my wife?"...or anything like that. He just stepped back and seemed to be grateful I was there to take over.

I whispered into her ear that it was time to let her mom go, hoping I wasn't sounding too goofy. It could have been that the mom and daughter had a bunch of unresolved issues. Maybe they fought a lot and had never made up? Or, maybe the daughter had never told her mom she loved her?...who knows?

But whatever, it was now too late for anything to happen that depended on two people communicating with each other.

The mom was on her way *out*, and this was the end of something.

As callous as it was, my job now was to get her to *clam up* and stop scaring all the other patients who were trying to sleep.

I was not really expecting it to work, but I suggested we step out of the room and move to the lounge where the soda machines were kept. Surprisingly to me, she responded to my gentle nudge as I pressed towards the door. Equally surprising, she also stopped screaming.

I did not know what I was doing, but *something* seemed to be working.

I couldn't believe it, but they were walking with me towards the lounge. The elevators were just across the hall and her husband suggested they go ahead and leave. That was the best thing I had heard so far because I had no idea what I was going to do next.

I shook his hand as they prepared to leave. Without saying anything, I reached over and just squeezed her arm as she continued to dab at her eyes with a soggy, white tissue.

He led her to the elevator and they were soon gone.

I breathed a deep sigh of relief. That was a scary one for me. If anyone had watched it all from a distance, it probably looked like I had done a good job. I honestly think she had cried herself out and was ready to be led away.

The janitor could probably have done the same thing.

Somehow, I had done something in there that seemed to make a difference to the grieving couple, but beats me what it was?

I ran into *stiff hair* in a hallway a couple of weeks later and she thanked me profusely for my help that night.

If she only knew.

IN HARM'S WAY

Public servants with *guns, badges* and *blue uniforms* were always present on Saturday nights.

After a while, I just expected to always see them hanging around in the hallways. The *objects* of their attention were usually in the trauma room. The officers always wanted to stay close to whomever they were associated with and did not want their *charge* to get out of sight.

One night, Nurse John casually asked me to escort a rather large and burly gentleman to the restroom as he submitted a urine specimen.

I thought my orders were a bit odd since the dude looked perfectly capable of urinating in the cup by himself. But I did as requested and made sure it happened properly.

As the large and burly gentleman was fastening his trousers in place, he asked what was going to happen to him next?

"Huh?"

I wasn't catching on.

He repeated the question and was wondering if *they* were going to take him away?

I still didn't get it.

I opened the door and we headed down the hallway to the triage station with the urine sample.

Just then, two armed and uniformed officers appeared around the corner. My rather large and burly friend instinctively turned and placed both hands against the wall while spreading his feet.

The officers quietly applied handcuffs to both my friend's wrists and led him outside to a patrol car. Evidently, an hour earlier, my new *friend* had rearranged the inside of a bar and sent several other patrons to another hospital.

I returned the urine sample to Nurse John.

I then asked John if maybe there was something he had forgotten to tell me about the patient I had just escorted to the bathroom?

…all by myself?

….like, don't turn your back on him or he might stick a knife between your ribs?

…or, be careful and don't let him take your head off?

…or, be careful that he doesn't poke your eyes out with a toilet plunger?

John just laughed and said the guy was harmless.

"Yeah, then why didn't YOU take him?"

I was learning about the *dark side* of being an ER, night volunteer.

PLAYING WITH TB

B ed "number one" in ERI was the only private room in ERI. Some patients were better off kept separate from the others.

One night I couldn't help but notice the hazard signs posted on the door with the cautionary labels to enter only with protective apparel.

The word **tuberculosis** caught my attention.

John asked me how I felt about going in there to gather the old Asian gal's vitals? I didn't mind. I knew about tuberculosis. It is a disease of the lungs that is transmitted through the air after the infected person coughed or sneezed. With the proper protection, I wasn't afraid of it.

Sally, one of the nurses with long blonde hair that reached almost to her waist, pulled me aside to get me properly *gowned.* I also needed a close-fitting mask to help filter out the *bad guys.*

I thought it might be sorta cool to go in there, even though I would be placing myself in harms way.

I could tell the guys about it back at the shop. I know it sounds stupid, but I found it exciting to be fighting dangerous bugs that could be a threat to mankind.

If I had been part of a medical team working in Africa, I would probably have been one of the first to go down from the deadly Ebola virus. That was just me.

It really wasn't a big deal. I gathered the gal's vitals as she slept... except for the temperature. I had to rouse her a bit to get the probe into her mouth. I just had to observe standard safety precautions and remove my protective garments while still in the room and place into a red bag with proper labeling.

I would tell my wife the following morning what I had been doing the night before and she would often take a couple of steps back... *quickly*.

HANDS

Early in my work, when I was still wearing a tie, we had a young guy come in...probably no more than sixteen years old who had both hands cut up really badly.

My brothers and I used to ask one another important questions that came into our heads, like:

"Which would you rather do, drown in a vat of snot?... or, slide down a rope of razor blades into a pool of alcohol?"

Well, this guy's hands looked like he had just slid down the *rope.*

I then noticed his *entourage* heading to the sidewalk outside.

Most of the guys were dressed in black with lots of leather and metal studs.

A couple of teen gals were included, one carrying a baby...about ten people, total. The patient did not want to follow the nurse's commands, and I am sure she also suspected he was a gang member.

I watched as she began *scrubbing* his raw and bleeding hands. It had to hurt like crazy. The kid was really fighting her, but it was the only way to clean the wounds and remove all the dirt. His hands really were sliced up badly and I couldn't imagine where a surgeon would even start to repair them.

After pouring an antiseptic over his hands....which I am also sure felt *wonderful*, she left him until the doctor could see him.

I stopped and chatted with him a little, but he didn't have much to say. I still wanted to treat him and his friends the same as anyone else, so I went outside to the sidewalk to chat with the others.

I suspect they thought I was going to harass them, as I suppose was often the case. But that was honestly not my plan.

I introduced myself as a volunteer and asked if there was any way I could assist them? One of the young guys stepped up real close to me...closer than we Angelo Saxon males normally get to one another here in America, and flipped my tie up, and into my face! I was surprised by that bold move, but tried not to show it.

It was like at the kitchen sink when returning the spray-hose to its holder with the water still running and accidentally spraying myself in the face. No harm done...just surprised and a bit startled.

I tried to act like this happened all the time and continued on with my *spiel.* I told him if there was anything I could do at all, I would be happy to help them.

At that, I returned to the building. I was called to deliver a urine sample to the lab, so I took care of that errand.

After returning, I passed the patient with the *hands* as he was walking out of ER I. I just assumed he needed to use the restroom. But instead of turning *left,* he turned *right*...for the door that led out to the sidewalk.

Two minutes later, his nurse came to me, asking where that patient had disappeared to?

"Beats me...but it looks like he's gone."

She and a couple of others frantically ran around looking for him...but he was nowhere to be found. That was the only time

I had ever seen a patient just get up and take off. Whatever his reasons, he decided he had had enough and *split*.

Many patients feel trapped once they are in the ER system while being serviced.

It is written in the *rules* that a person is free to leave at any time, but few ever do it. Most patients are there for their own good and are not inclined to leave before being dismissed.

But you *can* do it, and that teen was proof that once in a while, someone was indeed going to do it.

The thing that got my attention was the reaction from all the staff, as in...

"HOW DARE HE!"

But that's the way it works...no one can be held against their will and are free to walk out at any time.

THE WALKING DEAD

He looked like any other patient...mid-sixties male with his wife seated by his bed.

Right away, I sensed he was not the *talkative* type. He was direct with me and asked if his doctor was ready to talk with him yet?

He was sitting in the *full-Fowler* position....fully upright.

All he was doing was sitting upright. I guess someone had to place their *name* on that body-position so there would be no confusion as how to position a patient?

It sounds pretty arrogant to me. I guess some patients are better off seated in the *semi-Fowler* position, which would be sorta leaned back.

He coughed real hard a couple of times as I checked on the oxygen bottle underneath his gurney. I often checked on the oxygen bottle first, as though that was my main reason for stopping by. Most patients do not like it if they suspect I am stopping by just to talk to them specifically....still not sure why that is.

After making certain the bed had ample oxygen for use during a possible *transport*, I would ask how they were doing...using the same tone of voice my dad would use when wondering if it was going to rain that day.

He coughed hard again...but with a small amount of blood this time... into a white washcloth.

He asked if I did this with all the patients...checking on them?

I explained how I wanted to make sure everything was going okay with him. I sensed he wanted to shorten the conversation as he stared at me. He then informed me I was not going to be able to help him. His wife sat silently in her chair, not offering any input to the conversation.

I remained quiet...sensing he had something important he wanted to get off his chest. And he did indeed get right to the point as he disclosed his lung cancer, and how he knew he was going to die...real soon.

I then learned that he was also a medical doctor.

That was when my heart sank for him. He knew all the *ropes*, and all about what I was doing...or trying to do.

In my gut, I suddenly realized I was not going to help this man.

He had resigned himself to his fate and was probably only here in the ER because of insurance, or possibly at his wife's insistence.

It was a very hard moment for me as I knew there was nothing I was going to say to comfort him. I couldn't even joke about nurse *mustache* to distract him from his situation.

The attending ER doctor then came in to inform the patient-doctor of test results, and to make clear to him his options. The *attending* was straight with him and was being very matter-of-fact as he told him he did not have long, and that a refusal of treatment was his right.

The wife remained silent, seated in her chair.

The *attending* showed little emotion as they spoke. I was observing two professionals in conversation who knew exactly what they were talking about. I knew better than to offer any words of my own.

This guy was dying, and everyone knew it.

The patient-doctor then reached for his clothes and began to get dressed as his wife helped. I offered polite words of dismissal, like...

"Have a safe trip home."

His face was empty of emotion as he thanked me for the conversation. He was going to die soon, and no one on earth was going to stop that process.

I felt pretty useless just then.

I hate that feeling.

It happened one other time with a guy...maybe in his 40s who knew he was going to die soon.

He shared with me his frustration of having been seen by many doctors. He had been told there was nothing anyone could do for him. He knew he was going to die and *that* was *that*.

I must have tried to blot his situation out of my brain since I cannot even recall why he was dying.

After much thought, I decided on my response the next time it happens. My plan is to simply ask the patient if they are ready to die? If they want to confess their sins before God and ask forgiveness, I will help pray for them.

I decided that if they know they are *gone*, I will help them accept that and try to help them with the next step instead of feeling so helpless myself.

It happens to everyone at some point.

We might as well plan on it.

DEATH WATCH

As I came on duty one Saturday night, trauma room supervisor, John, grabbed me right away and had me sit with one of his patients. My orders were to sit and watch this mid-fifties guy and to call John if he were to suddenly croak.

This was my first time to be on a *death watch*.

John then filled me in on the details.

The mid-fifties male drove himself to the ER, saying he was having chest pains.

If you want to get a first-class seat up front, all you have to do is play the *chest pain* card. That will get you right up there....even ahead of the, *I just lost a finger* card.

The chest-pain guy got checked in, and then promptly *coded.*

I suppose I am a dunce, since I did not know for a long time exactly what it meant to *code.* There is even a "code room," which also took me a long time to get a handle on.

To all fellow dunces like myself, to *code* means your heart stopped, or your bodily processes stopped working to the point that you could be pronounced dead to the world.

This guy's heart had stopped twice before I had arrived, but they had brought him back each time. They had an EKG monitor on him, which would sound an alarm if he kicked off again, but John did not want to take any chances with this guy.

They had to use the *paddles* both times...and I'm not talking about a spanking.

He looked fine to me, sitting upright, smiling and talking. I introduced myself as we sat and chatted. He had no idea he had drifted off a couple of times into the great beyond. So far, he had not seen any *bright lights* at the end of a tunnel, so that was good news.

I kept my eye on him real hard, looking for anything unusual. He seemed to be like any other guy sitting at a bus stop waiting for a ride. I engaged him in regular conversation....my dog, kids, wife and work...the usual stuff.

He was a very regular guy, with the exception that he had one foot in the grave and the other on a banana peel.

The cardiologist on call was on his way to look at this guy. I was still at my post when he arrived...coming from sharing a dinner with friends at a local steak house.

Everyone "on call" must be within fifteen minutes of the hospital. But some of these surgeons must think all the other drivers on the road are going to pull over for them, because he was a long time in getting there. I know I sat there for thirty minutes before he arrived.

He must have been into a really good slice of chocolate cream pie.

But once there, he knew what needed to happen. This patient needed an emergency pacemaker...*stat.* That's medical-talk for, git-er-done-now.

Since I already had my own orders to be there, I stayed in place. After the cardiologist had checked him over, he ordered the necessary supplies to insert a wire into this guy's heart.

I knew this was a rare event, so I asked if I could stick around...you know, in case he needed someone to pass a scalpel, or something? And yeah, he was happy for me to stay and help. The cardiologist kept one nurse and ordered everyone else to clear out of the room...except for ME. I was now his *assistant.*

This was a cool step for me... automobile mechanic, ER volunteer, and now, assistant to the cardiologist. I was moving up in the world.

He explained his next moves to me so that we would be on the same page.

His plan was to insert a very long needle underneath the rib cage at the left, upper clavicle, and into the atrium of this guy's heart... a long reach. And the patient was to be awake the whole time... ouch!

My job was to keep his arms down, and to prevent him from jumping off the gurney!

The surgeon established a sterile field by applying the blue sterile towel with a hole cut out of the middle. He numbed the skin, and then pulled out what looked like a hallow knitting needle.

He told me to get a good grip, and began shoving the needle into this poor guy's chest, who might now wish he had dropped off earlier. I had to almost crawl on top of this guy to keep him on the gurney, but I kept him in place.

The surgeon was having trouble finding the *sweet spot* and kept hitting *something hard* with his dagger.

So he backed it out, and tried again. My head was almost in the patient's face as I worked to keep him still. This poor guy was really climbing the walls. I kept looking at him to see if the surgeon's work might push him over the edge?

He was shaking hard, but still with us.

The surgeon tried it a third time, but still just could not get his *sword* in the right place. So he finally decided to drop back and *punt*. He would move to the patient's neck and go down through the right jugular vein.

He explained to me that he normally did not like to go down through the neck, since the tubes would then be a real nuisance to the guy and hard to deal with.

I was really feeling sorry for this poor guy, having to endure someone stabbing him over and over while knowing it would not be polite to fight back. But I had to hand it to him, he was hanging in there and letting the surgeon work him over.

It reminded me of being on a double-date with my older brother as I sat in the back seat of his 1960 Ford Falcon. I thought it my duty to place my arm on the package shelf, *above* the shoulder of my date.

I don't remember if my arm was actually touching her, but I DO remember the blood draining out and losing all feeling in that arm as we rode for thirty minutes to the restaurant in Columbus, Indiana.

For some unknown reason, I had allowed myself to be tortured to the limits of human endurance...just like this poor guy.

From that point on, it was a piece of cake for the surgeon to run a wire down the patient's jugular vein and into his right atrium. With the wire hooked into the wall of the atrium, the temporary pacemaker could provide the electrical impulses to make his *ticker* do its job of making the blood move.

It was all very fascinating to me, and I was happy to have assisted in saving this man's life...however painful it must have been for him. He would now be stable until a permanent pacemaker could be surgically implanted into his chest to keep him alive for many years to come.

Of course, after that double-date, I went on to shoot myself in the foot many more times.

Unfortunately for me, there continues to be no known medical cure for my problem.

CLUMSY BIKERS

C rashing a motorcycle is usually not a lot of fun.
I once took a little trip through the air myself on my brother Mike's Yamaha 250.

I missed a turn, hit a driveway embankment and performed a *Walenda-type*, death-defying flying flip into a corn field. Fortunately for me, the field had just been plowed, so I had a semi-soft landing with no important parts broken...besides my pride.

Most bikers are not that fortunate.

We had them lined up in the hallway that night...two drug overdoses and one spousal abuse. Another pair of young and fit paramedics rolled the latest casualty into the trauma room. Our most recent daredevil was exiting a Dodgers ballgame with a little more speed than was appropriate.

I recall a favorite quote I had pinned to the wall above my toolbox back in the shop:

"Speed does not kill. It's usually the *stopping*"

And *stopping* is usually the tough part with biking.

Flying down the street at ninety miles per hour is a lot of fun... provided you are on an empty road in the middle of the desert. But this guy's road was far from empty with lots of cars and light poles on both sides.

I quickly delivered a box of gloves I had been sent for and headed into the double-door *chamber of horrors.* The surgeon and trauma-team Alpha were already into action as the lead paramedic filled everyone in on what they had found.

After the Dodgers had won their game, this guy was in a good mood and really nailed the throttle once he was on a street with a little room. They figured someone had changed lanes in front of him, forcing him straight into the back of a parked Buick Park Avenue. They estimated he was doing about *sixty* at the moment of impact.

As large-bore IV's were being inserted into his arms, others were cutting his clothes away. One of the paramedics casually explained to me what he usually saw with bikers after an unhappy, high-speed *stoppage* like this.

When the brain first gets a good handle on the situation, it begins a series of events to save itself. First, the hands are instructed to grip the handle bars with a force great enough to hold back a freight train.

The forearm bones usually snap first as the biker takes his or her *maiden flight* after coming into contact with a good old American-made bumper.

That would be the *ulna* and *radius* bones.

Those bones would often break in one, if not both arms.

But of course, that is not going to save the rider. The second thing the brain will do is...well, I guess that's *it*.

There are no other options.

It will be all up to the *hands and arms* to save the day.

If there is any time at all, a short prayer might be useful, but it will have to be quick...

"Dear God..." crunch!

As *said* rider begins his or her flight of freedom over the hardware, the legs always encounter difficulty in clearing the handlebars. The knee caps usually get the worst of it. They would catch on the bars, speedometer, tachometer, brake handles, mirrors, wobble-head dancers.... whatever is up there.

Once the knees clear the *table*, the lower legs usually then have enough room to follow. Although my paramedic friend said once in a while, a whole lower leg might come off if it caught just right. This guy seemed to be in luck since I thought I saw toes pointing up on *both* sides of the sheet.

If a rider is wearing a good helmet, most of his head might survive the impact with an automobile's windshield...the usual object in a rider's path. If no helmet is worn...all bets are off. There would be no hurry with *those guys* as a medic would then rummage through one of the cabinets for a body bag.

But even with a good helmet, there is still often brain and/or spinal cord damage.

This guy was commanding everyone's attention, so I stayed close in case they needed me to grab towels or something. I thought it was a shame they had to cut away this guy's nice, black leather riding jacket. But it was already torn in a couple of places on one arm.

His helmet was sitting on a chair against the far wall with a streak of silver paint injected into the cracked fiberglass. The face shield was nowhere to be seen. His riding pants were still intact, but also with dull streaks of silver paint in a couple of places. Bits and pieces of broken windshield safety glass fell from his jacket as it was pulled away.

Could he have hit a *silver* car?...duhh?

With all the clothing cut away, it was clear this guy's left kneecap had met with some resistance somewhere. It was resting a couple of inches lower on his leg than was customarily seen. His left arm also had an extra bend or two that were usually not seen in your average male form. He was also bleeding from several sites.

Broken bones are usually not that big of a deal unless they are poking into something important. The surgeon's real concern was with this guy's internal organs. He could be *bleeding out* underneath his covering of skin...something often overlooked by your average observer.

Of course the paramedics had applied a cervical collar to keep his head on straight. You don't want to inadvertently snap a spinal cord while checking for foreign objects on the backside.

With my new knowledge, I was very curious to see if this guy had all the injuries just described to me. But just then, this guy began vomiting. Every time he was moved, more ballpark franks and nachos made an egress from his stomach.

The paramedic explained that this guy most likely had some brain damage which caused the stomach to do its *thing* every time he was moved.

Watching someone vomit while lying on their back always makes me a little uncomfortable. I mean, it's going to come back down...right? And a guy has to breathe from that same hole... right?

This guy's blood pressure had dropped and the techs were having a tough time getting their needles into his collapsed veins. So everyone had their hands full. The surgeon then looked at ME and asked if I was comfortable with suctioning his airway?

ALLRIGHT....I was ready to go!

I knew how to do this and was happy to be put to work.

I grabbed the suction hose and began clearing out his pie-hole. I knew from my EMT training to not also suction out all his air at the same time. And every time the radiologists moved him the least little bit...there went Old Faithful again!

It was not long before the X-rays were ready and thrown onto the illuminated screen on the wall. From my position ten feet away, even I could see that both bones of his left forearm were adequately broken....the *radius* and *ulna*.

The surgeon seemed to think the left leg bones were intact, but the kneecap, or *patella,* was torn from its usual spot. That would be the tendon of the *quadriceps femoris* muscle...one of the big muscles in the front of your thigh.

By now, our subject's stomach was mostly empty, and with only the dry heaves. I was still at my post, but things were quieting down. The surgeon alerted radiology that we would soon need to get an MRI on this guy.

They still wanted me at my post, so the portable suction unit was hooked to the gurney. I enjoyed being included with the trauma team and was feeling good about being put to use.

I no longer said much to the guys back at the shop during morning break about what I had been doing the previous Saturday night.

Had I told them exactly what I had been doing, they probably would not have believed me anyway.

We hurried this guy to the elevator and up one floor to radiology. There was always a ton of equipment to transfer to the MRI table with a patient like this. All of us workers had to get in the booth with the operator and away from the powerful magnetic beams.

A neurosurgeon had been called to check on this guy. We usually did not see those guys just yet, but he was already close by and wedged his way into the control booth with us to view this guy's brain. It was always fascinating to watch the slices of brain and skull come up on the screen as the electron beam made its passes.

It was hard for me to tell for sure what I was looking at until I saw the eyeballs. As more of the brain showed up, the surgeon began pointing out what he always looked for. He noted some small white places on the scan which indicated *bleeds* from broken vessels. He instructed all of us how to look for abnormal things on one hemisphere that might not be the same as on the opposite side.

Since this guy had been wearing a good helmet, there was no obvious skull deformation. The surgeon said this type of injury usually healed by itself and would not need his intervention. The *bleeds* all seemed to be small. They would have to monitor his condition and see how he progressed.

After the expensive *photo session*, we rolled him back down to the trauma room. A *bone surgeon* had been called and was ready to take him into surgery. Our patient was awake and answering questions, so that was all very good. He was looking better all the time.

The Orthopedic surgeon explained to the patient how he would open up his knee and wire the cap back into place, as well as operating on his arm to put those bones back together. It looked like this guy was going to pull through after all. And I was there to help.

I was remembering a "Shake-and-Bake" TV commercial from my youth (bread mixture to coat chicken) where a little kid would announce at the end,

"...and ah hay-oped,"...in a down-south accent.

I wanted to announce the same thing...

"Yes, I helped."

It felt good to have helped save this guy's life...me, the ER volunteer.

BRAIN BUCKETS

The paramedics were really straining to move this three-hundred-pound biker to a hospital gurney in the trauma room.

He wore a black leather vest, jeans, brown cowboy boots and sported a heavy silver chain around his neck. When they removed the chain, I was almost expecting to see a boat anchor attached to one end.

He had tattoos in abundance on his chest and arms, with gray streaks in his long beard and equally long gray hair.

This guy was a die-hard biker who had *dropped* his Harley.

The paramedics described what they had found. Evidently, another biker in the group had unexpectedly stopped quickly at a traffic light in front of this guy and he lost his balance, falling over and hitting his head on the curb.

This was not the result of a high-speed collision or death-defying stunt...just a simple, falling-over-and-landing-on-the-ground... *bump*. He was barely moving at the time.

The paramedic also explained that the biker complained of being unable to see out of his right eye. He had some *road rash* on his right arm, but appeared to be unhurt otherwise.

I noticed a frown creep over our trauma surgeon's face as he examined this guy.

He mentioned aloud that he suspected nerve damage somewhere in this guy's head. I saw him then get on the phone to the operator to see if a specialist was near?

As luck would have it, a crack-neurosurgeon was indeed close by...only ten minutes away, playing basketball in a gym. They placed the call and he was on his way.

While we waited, the paramedic began explaining to me why this guy's injuries were so bad. He picked up the *helmet* and explained how the *German-style, WWII* helmet was for *looks only* and worthless for protecting a biker's head.

He said the paramedics called them, "brain buckets."

After a crash, all they were good for was holding a biker's brains.

I examined the black, cheaply-made helmet and agreed. California has a law requiring all motorcyclists to wear helmets, but each rider has his choice of helmet. The German-style helmet was worn by the guys who were passively protesting the fact that they were being forced to wear a helmet in the first place.

This guy had made his choice, and was now in danger of losing sight in one eye.

The neurosurgeon was there rapidly. I grabbed a clean apron for him to wear, covering his white T-shirt, blue gym shorts and white Nike *sneaks*. After examining the patient, the neurologist determined this guy was suffering from a type of compartment syndrome where he had burst blood veins and swelling, which was putting pressure on the optic nerve.

He said he could often save most of a patient's sight if he could get the proper meds in him within *two hours* of the incident. He would also need to open up the injured area with a scalpel to try and relieve some of the pressure.

The paramedic said we were at, "one hour and forty minutes."

The trauma surgeon got on the phone to the pharmacy at the other end of the hospital...

...and I got ready.

Making emergency runs to the pharmacy fell under MY jurisdiction.

I watched the trauma surgeon carefully as he placed the order. While still talking on the phone, he looked in my direction and lifted one eyebrow...that was my signal.

I was off like a shot.

My special friend, nurse *Mud Face*, had filled me in on how the pharmacy worked at night when everything else was closed down. When an order was called in from ER, they would pull the required meds and place them in the curved, stainless steel trough at the base of the thick, safety glass.

At first, I didn't think she was serious. I mean, *anyone* could come by and pick up these meds....couldn't they? Evidently, they did not see that as a problem, since security was there and no one else should know about it late at night. The pharmacy staff knew someone from ER would be there right away, and did not want to be bothered answering the "night bell."

My first time to do this, I rang the bell anyway, not quite believing the hospital was this trusting. And sure enough, the pharmacist was annoyed at my having rung the bell....

"It's, *right there.*"

But I decided on my own that it might be possible that *two* doctors could be ordering meds at the same time, and I wanted to be sure I was getting the right stuff. So I always made sure I asked questions and knew *who* was sending me, and exactly *what* I was supposed to be getting.

Joseph Apple

I ran to the heavy safety glass, reach down, and it was right there…
a vial of special medication that might save this biker's eyesight.
I grabbed it and resumed my mad dash back to the trauma room.
Time was of the essence.

A set of heavy double-doors separated the Emergency Department from the remainder of the hospital, with a big sign that
read,

"Emergency Department, Authorized Personnel Only."

I had the codes for all the doors in the hospital and the signs were
no longer a novelty to me. I was as *authorized* as it got.

I rapidly punched in the code and continued on my way as the
doors slowly crept open for me. I don't dare share the codes with
anyone because they are probably still the same. They never
change them.

I made my trip in about two minutes…they had thirteen more to
save an eye.

I handed over the vial and the neurosurgeon began his injections.
I stepped back and watched as he grabbed his scalpel and carefully made a long incision above the biker's eye.

He continued his careful cutting, about the way my younger
brother David trims fat from a piece of round steak. David does
not like the feel of fat in his mouth, and I am sure he could have
performed this part equally as well.

The surgeon carefully made small cuts until reaching the damaged area without disrupting other vital nerves and vessels. More
blood spurt out as the *logjam* was relieved. The neurosurgeon
then kept the wound open and watched it carefully as he dabbed
at it with 4x4, sterile gauze pads. He calmly explained to our
trauma surgeon what should happen and what to expect next.

Our trauma surgeon was always *boss* with the patients who came through this room. But it was clear that he was stepping back to let the *expert* handle this one.

The biker was in good hands.

Hey, *my* hands were in there too, huh?

How about that.

TOO CLOSE TO HOME

I was all showered, dressed in my burgundy scrubs and blue volunteer jacket, ready to head for the door when I heard a horrific crash outside on the street. We often heard crashes at our intersection, but nothing like what I had heard this time.

This one was heavy-duty.

I instinctively reached in my pocket to make sure I had gloves, and headed for the door. From the sound of the crash, it had to be bad.

As I opened the door, there were no cars at our intersection, but rather in the middle of the block. It was dark out just then. I ran on out to see a 30's gal walking in the street and screaming a lot. Her blue Chrysler minivan was in one of my neighbor's yards with the left front smashed all the way back to the windshield.

An older, red Toyota was sitting in the middle of the street with an equally smashed left front. But the driver was still in the car and not moving much. I assumed the gal's minivan had an air bag that had inflated, saving her from serious injury. The driver of the older Toyota was not so fortunate.

He appeared to be an Asian male…maybe in his thirties, wearing a blue T-shirt and jeans. He looked like any other regular guy.

As I ran to his door, he seemed to be pinned in place. Most likely, his feet and legs were smashed in the floor pan of his crumpled car as I had seen happen so many times to those brought into the trauma room where I spent my Saturday nights.

I quickly noticed the steering wheel was badly twisted. In cases such as this, I knew how important it was to keep a patient's head and neck stable to prevent further damage to the spinal cord at the cervical spine.

The car had four doors, so I yanked on the left rear door and climbed inside. I asked if he understood me? I checked him over quickly for any massive bleeding, but did not see anything. He mumbled something in another language, so I had no idea if he spoke English. I announced that I was going to hold his head until help arrived. He mumbled again, but it was gibberish.

My neighbors were coming out of their houses.

Someone yelled that they had called 911. Someone else was in the street to stop traffic. Porch lights were coming on all around as the gal from the mini-van continued her wandering and screaming.

I soon heard the sirens of rescue vehicles on their way. Our street had a slight bend right here, and it looked as though the minivan had crossed the centerline, crashing headlong into this poor guy in the Toyota.

As the firemen arrived, I identified myself as an EMT and told them what I was doing. They had me stay in place as they surveyed the scene. They decided they would need their Jaws-of-Life to pry the metal apart to get this guy out.

Once they had their equipment set up, another fireman took my place to prevent anything from happening to me. At that point, my work was finished. I had done all I could do.

Before long, there was a whole mass of people out in the street with TV news crews showing up as well. Our block had been cordoned off and all traffic diverted to side streets.

As I watched the situation unfold, I overheard an officer mention how the gal in the minivan had tested *positive* for alcohol. That would explain her misjudging the slight bend in the road at the end of our block. She was probably also going too fast, as many drivers often did on our street at night.

It took at least thirty minutes to extricate the Asian male and get him into an ambulance. By the time they got him to a hospital, they would be pushing the envelope of the *golden hour* in which to save a severely injured victim.

I had my EMT certification, but had never really used it in employment. I earned it for my own medical knowledge for just this type of situation. I had been near medical emergencies in the past and hated the helpless feeling of not knowing what to do.

I had done the right thing, but there really was not much I or any other bystander could have done.

After the dust had settled, I continued on to my post in the ER for that Saturday night. I asked around to see if the victim had been brought to *my* hospital, but he must have been taken somewhere else.

This was one more example of the carnage caused by someone who had thoughtlessly jumped into an automobile after having consumed an alcoholic beverage. If only the drinking drivers could see what their actions caused *before* committing this crime? And it certainly is a crime.

There was nothing humorous about this incident...nothing at all.

Once all the glass and twisted metal had been removed and the street flushed clean, little trace of the accident remained. I later noticed on my walks bits of yellow plastic from a parking lamp lens and shards of shiny plastic molding at the curb. These tell-tale indicators could be found at most any street-side curb.

And the Asian male who had been innocently driving to the grocery store that night?

I later learned from a neighbor he had died.

MERRY-GO-ROUND

I was really proud of myself.

I could watch the trauma surgeon cut open a chest and it did not bother me at all. I was now able to look at patients as though they were cars or trucks and not real people.

When first exposed to blood and needles in the ER, I wasn't sure if I could handle this. I always hated to have a needle sink deep into my arm, and it was even worse to watch it.

As I made my rounds one night, I saw a guy on a gurney in ER II who seemed to be about my age. I introduced myself as usual to see if he wanted some company. He did seem to want to talk, so I settled in with him to help him pass the time.

I had learned long ago that few patients ever wanted to talk about their injury or physical problem, so I never asked. And there was often a long wait as the lab processed blood work.

And this guy was no different. We talked as though we had met in a diner and wondering if the Dodgers were going to make it to the Series this year?

Eventually, he began talking about his wife and how things were not going so well. He mentioned how he had lost his job and was trying to find work. He seemed more relaxed as we talked and he decided to let me in on why he was there.

He held up one arm to reveal a long gash across that arm, near his wrist.

I figured this guy was really having a bad day to cut himself in his shop to add to all his other problems. He seemed to enjoy my hanging out with him, so I continued talking about whatever came to mind...volcanoes, earthquakes and other things I enjoyed reading about.

But he kept coming back to how lousy things were at home and how he did not have answers for so many things.

Then, finally, he held up his *other* arm to reveal a similar gash near that wrist.

It hit me like a brick in the head...he had tried to commit suicide.

This changed everything. I no longer felt like I was working on a Volkswagen bug. This guy was a living, breathing human being with problems so bad he wanted to end it all.

I placed one hand on his shoulder and tried to communicate to him how badly I felt for him. He was now starting to really get into it and began sharing the details of his ordeal.

His wife had been yelling at him in the kitchen and even smashed a plate on the floor. She was mad about the bills and thought he was not trying hard enough to find another job.

I began having a funny feeling in my head.

He continued by telling me how he went to the bathroom and threw the soap dispenser against the tile wall above the tub. He then began looking for a razor blade, but could not find one.

I felt my face starting to tingle.

But he did notice his safety razor on a shelf and realized it had a couple of sharp blades inside the plastic head. He described to me how he had to stomp on it several times with the heel of his shoe to get the tiny blades out.

He said it was really difficult to remove those blades without slicing his fingers. But once he had them out, he did what he had in mind to do.

Suddenly, I knew I needed to sit down.

My *Merry-go-round* was taking off.

At first, I did not realize what was happening to me?

Why was I feeling like this?

It wasn't the gashes…at least not the *first* one.

Why was my head starting to spin like this? Why am I about to keel over? This did not make sense to me. But I for-sure knew I needed to sit before I *fell*. I quickly excused myself and left.

I don't remember what I said and hoped I did not say something stupid like:

"Well, good luck with all that."

As I sat on a box of toilet paper rolls in the supply closet, I tried to sort it all out.

My *merry-go-round* was slowing down, but still spinning faster than I wanted. I could feel my blood returning to my head. I had been volunteering in the ER for several years now, so this sort of thing should not have affected me like this. It just did not make sense to me.

What was it about this guy that caused me to start spinning again?

And then it slowly dawned on me. Instead of seeing this guy as a *telephone pole*, I had begun seeing him as a neighbor, or a brother.

I found myself *caring* for him.

I still cared for all the patients, but this one caught me off guard.

I knew how only a slight breeze might make my *Merry-to-round* start spinning. I suppose I was working hard to suppress any real feelings I might have about a person's pain where blood was involved.

I was indeed proud of myself for conquering that supposed *flaw* in myself that caused me to spin out of control so easily. But this guy changed things. I realized I was not in control at all...at least, not if I *really* cared.

I continued with my work. There were more messy gurneys to wipe down and get ready. I still was not feeling so hot and just wanted to do some grunt-work. I was not ready to talk to patients any more just then. I did not put it together all at once...it took a while.

I still had to work at it to keep my *Merry-go-round* still and not spinning out of control. I had to find a balance between seeing the patients as real people and not tree trunks. I think most of the nurses had to look at them as *tree trunks*. Otherwise, they would not be able to do their jobs.

With a lot of practice, I learned how to stay in touch with patients and their pain without falling in a heap. But I found it to be like disarming a bomb without getting blown to smithereens...a delicate task.

It was a tough job to stick my head right down in there and mess with all those funny wires and tricky switches without blowing things up...and blowing myself up.

After finding a measure of success with the *playground equipment*, I finally hit on a balance that worked *most* of the time...but not *all* of the time.

So how would I know when I was doing it right and really in touch with a patient?

You would find me in the supply closet, sitting on a box of toilet paper rolls with my head between my knees *dragging my feet in the dirt* while trying to get this thing to slow down.

WHEN FOOD IS THE BEST MEDICINE

I had just come on duty, and as usual, poked my head in the trauma room to see if anything really good was happening.

John, the trauma room supervisor was tending to an old guy who gave no immediate indication as to why he was there.

A patient had to satisfy certain criteria to be treated in the trauma room.... gunshot wound... knife wound... automobile accident...fall from a roof...those sorts of things. I was curious, so I stepped to his bedside to get the story.

I loved it when John was on duty because he used me a lot...as though I was his assistant.

Right away, he asked me to gather this guy's vital signs. I got busy with getting his blood pressure, temperature, blood oxygen level, heart rate and respiration count. I tried talking to him, but he could only mumble things that made no sense.

At first I suspected this guy was a stroke victim. But John thought it might be something else. I asked his name, and instead of acting real lethargic, he was very animated with his gestures and trying really hard to explain things to me.

I asked if he knew what day this was? And after thinking for a couple of seconds, he muttered something that sounded like *Saturday*...which was right.

But his speech was all out of sync and sounded disjointed. And again, he really sounded like a stroke victim.

I recalled playing a game with my sisters where we would hold our tongues with a thumb and index finger and try talking that way. Everyone else had to guess what we were saying.

My sisters were older than me and I was new to the game. They instructed me to hold my tongue and repeat the words:

"I'm an apple."

They then laughed at me real hard as I tried my best.

I didn't get it.

Mom yelled at them to knock it off.

And that was how this guy sounded...like he was holding his tongue with his fingers. It sounded like he was trying to tell me something important, but I could not figure it out. I guess a neighbor saw him lying on the sidewalk in front of their condo and called paramedics.

John withdrew some urine from the catheter bag and ran a dip-test to check his urine glucose level. It was a bit high, so John was wondering if maybe this guy's insulin production might be out of whack? I think John had seen this before with diabetics, but this was the first time for me. This guy looked like he was in pretty bad shape.

John then sent me to get a box-lunch for this guy.

We always kept box-lunches in small refrigerators in each ER section. Most of the time, the ER fridges were empty. That was one of the *grunt-jobs* I could always do, since few nurses had the time to do it.

It was good old *Mud Face* who first showed me how to do it.

She took me to the cafeteria, going through the rear service entrance to one of the big walk-in refrigerators. She instructed me to always give a yell to see if anyone was there. If no one was around, I was to then help myself and load up several box lunches for both of our ER refrigerators.

That was one more task I could do that made me feel useful around there. And the nurses were always happy to see me do it.

I learned that some of the nurses would help themselves to the lunches when no one was looking. Mud Face said they were not supposed to do it, but it still happened. They would not want to be seen with one of the green-and-white boxes, so they would just rob a sandwich or bag of chips.

No one ever took the apple.

I rolled a tray over the lap of our senior patient and removed the cellophane from the ham and cheese sandwich. I also opened the box of orange juice and shoved a straw into the container.

His hands jerked a lot, but he was able to get the sandwich to his mouth to take a bite. I helped guide the straw to his mouth as he took a sip.

While he worked on that, I got busy cleaning the other gurney there in the trauma room. John then explained to me this guy had been brought to the trauma room because he had been found on a sidewalk and no one knew if he had fallen, or what?

John also explained that often, some of the older dudes would forget to eat and then their system would start acting funny.

As I worked, I slowly noticed that his speech was beginning to clear up. John noticed it as well. He was quite verbal, and we were able to understand more of that he was saying.

Pretty soon, he was talking as clearly as anyone else with a mouth full of food.

Clearly, this was the most dramatic recovery I had ever seen in the ER. His glucose levels had fallen enough that his brain was not firing on all cylinders.

Once we had him *re-fueled,* he was ready to hit the track for a few more laps.

I learned a good medical lesson with that patient. Just because something *walks* like a duck and *quacks* like a duck does not mean it is a duck.

Sometimes it is only someone in need of a *quacker* (please forgive me).

NURSE NUTS-O

I had just finished restocking the blanket heater with a fresh load of blankets when I noticed a commotion with a patient going into the private room.

Patients who were causing problems were often placed in the private room. And sure enough, this gal was yelling and cursing at the nurses who were rolling her around.

I was curious.

As a volunteer, I enjoyed the unique freedom of not having anything I absolutely *had* to do and was free to roam around. I had tasks to perform, like keeping the bedside cabinets restocked and making up the gurneys, but I was an *extra*.

My most important job was to just **be there**. Whenever a nurse would remark aloud:

"Hey, do we have anyone to....?"

That would usually be ME.

And as I poked my head into the private room, nurse *big eyelashes and cleavage* asked if I could stay with this patient and keep an eye on her?

"Sure, no problem."

That was what I was there for.

The first thing I noticed was the *leather restraints* on the 30's female patient's wrists that kept her hands secured to the side railings.

From my training, I knew that securing a patient to a gurney was a serious issue and had to come straight from the ER doctor-in-charge.

This gal looked fine to me, so I was wondering why she was acting so violently that she needed to be tied down? I did not smell alcohol, which usually explained everything.

I began talking to her in an attempt to get her to calm down. My soft voice often worked on patients such as this who were scared of the hospital.

I began by asking her name and how she was feeling? She responded by loudly asking if I was here to pull her teeth?

"No, I am not here to pull your teeth."

She then asked if I was going to suck her brains out her ears?

"Hmmmmm"

"No, I am not going to mess with your ears...or the stuff behind them."

She then asked if I would take the picture off the wall and to please make *the guys* on the ceiling leave the room?

"OKAY......Now I get it."

"We've got a *nutso* here."

I had no idea how to get the *guys* on the ceiling to leave, so I said they looked friendly enough to me, and could they please stay? To sound more believable, I said one was a good friend of mine and I wanted him to stick around.

She reluctantly relented and said they could stay...as long as they kept their mouths shut.

I told her I would jump on them at the first hint of trouble, which seemed to satisfy her.

She then noticed my blue volunteer jacket and asked how long I had been volunteering, and did I enjoy my work?

I thought, "What?"

That last sentence made sense…what gives here?

This was now starting to get a little spooky. I then asked her about herself and what sort of work she did?…not knowing what in the world to expect from that sort of normal question? I was not expecting her to be working *anywhere.*

But she surprised me by saying she had worked for many years as a nurse, but was currently unemployed.

Just then, her nurse entered our room to gather her vitals.

The *nutso* gal then began yelling and screaming at the top of her lungs, saying that nurse was not about to touch her with those filthy, germy hands.

The nurse tried talking calmly to her, saying she was just going to gather her blood pressure.

"Not with those long fingernails, you're not!" she screamed.

I looked, and sure enough, the nurse had very long, painted fingernails.

"Did you wash your hands before you came in here?" she screamed again.

The nurse did not answer.

"And don't you know you are supposed to keep your fingernails short?" she queried. She continued with, "You've got millions of germs underneath those dirty fingernails!"

I thought to myself..."Boy, she's right!"

This gal really should not have those long fingernails. They taught us these things in my EMT classes.

The nurse then wrapped the cuff around the patient's arm and gathered the blood pressure anyway. Our *nutso* patient did not have much choice about it with her wrists secured to the bed rails.

Patient *Nutso* was not about to open her mouth for the temperature probe, so the attending nurse left.

Nutso directed her wrath back to me again and asked if I would *please* get those guys off the ceiling?...she did not trust them up there.

"No, No...I really want them to stay," I responded.

I mean, how am I going to get them out?...and how will I know when they are gone?"

And if someone were to come into the room while I was *sweeping* the ceiling with a broom...who's nutso then?

I tried to steer her back to her earlier comment about working as a nurse.

She said she had worked for many years as an orthopedic nurse in a major hospital in Arizona before coming to California. For some reason, she also mentioned that she had been fired from her last job. As she opened up, I suspected she was beginning to trust me.

I glanced *up* to see if the *guys* on the ceiling were behaving themselves...which they seemed to be doing.

She was settling down as she continued about how she had free access to all the pain meds in the hospital where she last worked. She confided that she would often help herself to the really strong stuff they kept in there.

It was all beginning to make sense to me now. This gal had fried her brain on drugs.

But she wasn't *completely* gone.

I mean, she was absolutely right about the nurse with the long fingernails. Those long red fingernails with the silver stars most likely harbored some nasty critters under there. I couldn't blame her on that one.
She then suddenly jerked her head around and asked what was flying around in our room?

"I don't know...don't make me guess...a bat?"

"No silly, she replied...I think it's a fly."

Ahhh, now she's got *me* doing it.

So I went ahead and asked her how the *guys on the ceiling* were getting along?

She said they were all asleep in their chairs.

Whew...I was glad of that. I was not sure how much more of this I could take.

Just then, two EMTs entered our room from CMH with their own gurney. If you need to ask, that's *County Mental Health.*

They buckled her in and carted her off...kicking and screaming.

I had heard about nurses who had wasted themselves on drugs available to them in a hospital, but this was my first time to witness it first-hand. The sad thing was, *part* of her was here, and the rest was off in la-la-land somewhere.

But honestly, it was sad. She had destroyed herself and would never be the same.

I was really shaking my head after that patient. That was a new experience for me to witness a mixture of reality and drug-induced mental illness.

Before leaving the private room, I figured I should go ahead and wipe down the gurney and apply clean sheets.

Upon exiting the room, the guys on the ceiling called out and asked if I would please turn the light off before leaving?

...which I did.

OLD LADIES

I was tired this night and did not want to get too heavily involved in anything.

After a busy Saturday of working on my car, cleaning the garage and working on the sprinkler system in our front yard, I was just pooped.

I was doing simple things...running to the lab...gathering gurneys and changing oxygen bottles. I didn't really want to get too involved with any of the patients.

But as I walked through ER I, I had the odd sensation I should stop and talk to this one old gray-haired gal.

I saw them often...elderly women who were usually in lots of pain. Most of them did not want to be bothered, and I really did not feel like taking the chance.

I had already walked past her bed twice without stopping. But a little voice inside my head kept annoying me by reminding me that this was one of my big reasons for working in the Emergency Department.

So I decided to ignore the *bad angel* on my left shoulder and listen to the *good angel* on my right shoulder.

As I walked to the side of her bed, she then opened her eyes and forced a faint smile. I introduced myself as a volunteer and inquired about how she was feeling? She sat up a little and said she was in a lot of pain, but did not disclose the nature of her pain.

I realized right away maybe she wanted to talk after all. I never knew what would work, so I usually began by talking about my own day and what I had been doing.

Our daughter was making a Pinewood Derby race car from balsa wood that the parents were supposed to help with. So I told her all about that and how I had cut out a figure of a surfer on a band saw my daughter had drawn for me.

My daughter's idea was to mount a surfer on top of the *car* which was shaped like a *wave* with the surfer on a surfboard. I would have never thought of something like that for a car. It was a cool idea.

The old gal seemed to cheer up as I spoke. She added how she had always loved to work with her hands in building projects. I also mentioned working in the yard that afternoon and repairing a broken sprinkler head. And she joined in with how much she loved to work in the dirt with flowers and plants.

We were beginning to really connect and hit it off. She had a nice smile and seemed to understand how I thought. So I kept going and added how I enjoyed writing and how the English language was always evolving. She agreed with me and spoke of the news articles she had written for her alma mater.

This was a gal I could really spend some time with.

After a while, I was forgetting that she was here because of a painful ailment.

We talked for over an hour. I could usually tell when someone was talking just to be *courteous*, but she seemed to really enjoy my company...and I hers.

Before long, her nurse came to take her to X-ray and to run some tests. I was needed in other places as well. But I did enjoy visiting with her, even though I would not see her again. She was just a nice person to spend time with.

Normally, that would have been the end of things.

The reason I am even mentioning her is that two weeks later, I received a copy of a letter in my box at the volunteer office. This gal's adult daughter had taken the time to write a letter to a hospital administrator thanking me for spending time with her mother.

They were vacationing from Arizona when her mom suddenly began developing severe abdominal pains. It was discovered she had a kink in her colon which required surgery. She had been in great pain and was very frightened to be having this problem far from home.

She went on to describe *me*, and how special it was that I had taken the time to sit with her mom and help get her mind off her pain. She went on and on about me...blah, blah, blah...and all that, and what a wonderful hospital this was to care about the patients like this.

I thought, well, okay. That's good. That's what I'm here for. I was happy to have helped her.

I suppose it all looked great on the outside, but they couldn't see what I was thinking before stopping to check on her.

They did not know that it was by only the thinnest of margins that I had stopped to spend time with her. I really was not feeling up to it that night. I suppose it was good that the hospital looked good through what I had done.

But I know that sort of thing goes both ways. There were probably other patients there that same night who had terrible experiences while this one went well.

When you go to the Emergency Department, it is often a *crap shoot.* You never know how it is going to turn out in even the best of hospitals.

I decided it was best that I was conducting myself the way I was... just for me. Maybe I had helped that gal, but on that particular night, she had returned the favor and helped me just as much.

I thought this was the way things should be working.

Oh, and our daughter's Pinewood Derby car? She did not win a race, but she did win an award for overall, "Best Design!"

"And ah hay-oped."

FUN WITH ALZHEIMER'S

A t first, I did not see it.

This old gal looked just like the many other gray-haired gals I had spent time with. She had a narrow face with neatly styled hair and a nice smile. After introducing myself, I engaged her in conversation to help her pass the time.

I noticed she had a bloody bandage wrapped around her left hand which she was constantly picking at. She had partially pulled it away and I could see that she had a three-inch gash across that hand at the base of her fingers. She did not volunteer the information on how it had happened, so I did not ask.

I asked about her level of pain and added that it must really hurt? But she did not mention her pain at all. Instead, she began talking about her daughter, Shirley, who was still at home with their collie, Dutchess.

I added that we also had a dog, a Husky named Corky.

She made no mention of a husband, but added that she lived in a yellow, three-story house on Oak Street that had lots of red tulips by the driveway. I added that I also loved red tulips and how I used to get in trouble for picking them when a child.

She nervously picked at her bandage a bit more, and I advised her she should probably not bother it until the doctor had looked at it.

She then added that she had a daughter, Shirley, who was home with their collie, Dutchess.

I thought, *another* daughter named Shirley?

She continued with her descriptions of the yellow house and the red tulips along the driveway.

It was all beginning to sound *vaguely familiar* to me!

Didn't she just say all of this?

She seemed quite normal…up to that point. But her smile and genuineness did not betray her. I sensed she really believed all she was saying, and did not realize she was repeating herself.

At that point, I realized this gal must have Alzheimer's and was stuck in a conversational loop.

Just then, her nurse dropped by and pulled me aside.

She confirmed my suspicions about this gal's dementia and asked if I would stay with her and prevent her from yanking at her bandage. She added that the old gal had pushed her hand through a window at the nursing home and would need stitches.

The ER doctor was quite busy and could not get to this gal for a while yet.

Of course, I agreed to do whatever I could. I was always impressed when the nurses asked for my help. I had the time to sit with her… something they could not do. So I pulled up a chair to see where this would go?

She was just beginning to tell me about her daughter, Shirley… *again*. So I stopped and asked how old Shirley was?

She replied, "*four.*"

"Okay."

So I dug a little deeper and asked what color hair Shirley had?

She responded that Shirley had beautiful, long blonde hair.

"Okay, go on."

So she began explaining how *Shirley* was home with their collie, *Dutchess.*

I asked about the coloring of *Dutchess?*

She replied that *Dutchess* was brown and white, with a round white patch on her forehead.

"Okay, continue."

She then proceeded to describe their yellow, three-story house on Oak Street.

I asked if they had a porch swing?

She responded that they did indeed have a porch swing that would hit against the house if they swung too hard, scratching the paint. She continued by describing their lovely red tulips along the driveway.

I stopped her nurse as she passed and asked if it would be *long* before the doctor would be seeing this gal? She told me to get *comfortable* since a heart attack victim had just been rolled in.

I sensed I was in for a long night.

My charge for the night then began a *new* conversation about her *daughter* at home with their *dog.*

I was beginning to get a little bored with this, so I interrupted her and said,

"Wait a minute, is your daughter's name, Shirley?"

"Why yes! How did you know?"

"Ahhh, lucky guess?"

"And I'll bet she is four years old and has long, blonde hair?"

"Why that's amazing...how did you know that?"

And so she continued with the dog.

This was too much fun, so I kept at it.

I interrupted again: "Tell me...your dog...by any chance was it a brown and white *collie?*"

"Why, you are indeed a genius," she added. "Yes, it was."

"And did it have a patch of *white* on its forehead?"

By this time she thought I was "Marvin the Magnificent."

She continued about the *yellow house.*

And of course, I had to ask if she had a *porch swing* that would bump the house when they rocked too hard, scratching the paint?

She seemed unduly amazed that I knew every detail of her life.

And before long, we were on the same loop again...over and over.

This was great fun, but even so, I was beginning to get bored again.

Finally, the ER doctor was able to get to her.

He noticed that I had her well contained, and asked if I would mind changing into sterile gloves and continue keeping her occupied while he worked on her hand?

"Sure, why not?"

So, one of the nurses fixed me up with a pair of size ten, sterile gloves.

The doctor was seated on a stool and out of view from the old gal, so I explained to her what "I" would be doing. I was not sure what she could understand, but thought I owed it to her to explain what would be taking place.

Once the doctor had cleaned and established a sterile field around the hand, I explained to her she would feel a few stabs of pain from the needle as the pain killer was injected. Even though she might not be able to comprehend what I was saying, I thought it was an injustice when doctors explained the pain as a *pinch*.

It *never* feels like a *pinch*.

It *always* feels like a stab from a needle.

I was holding her arm to keep it steady, and she tried to jerk away with the first couple of pokes. So I spoke again...

"Oh, I'm sorry. Did that hurt? I will try to be more careful."

Of course I knew she would no longer be feeling it in a couple of minutes.

The doctor did not say anything to me, but just smiled.

And he continued with stitching her hand to put her back together as I steadied her arm.

I turned to the old gal as he worked and continued asking about her *daughter, dog, house and flowers*? But I stopped playing *Marvin the Magnificent,* since the doctor was right there. He might not appreciate my *bedside manner*.

However, when finished, he did look me directly in the eye and say,

"Thanks."

That was as good as it usually got from one of the doctors. And I understood it fully.

Joseph Apple

Before leaving the bedside, I patted the old gal on the shoulder and advised her to not swing *too* hard on the porch swing so that it would not hit the house and scratch the paint.

"Why, how did you know?"

ON A SERIOUS NOTE

When I first began volunteering in the ER, the helicopter helipad was just outside the ER in one portion of the parking lot.

All the old nurses knew to not park near the fence, or else they would wind up with stone chips on their windshields from prop wash. And once again, it was good ole *Mud Face* who filled me in on the hazards of parking over there.

I am certainly indebted to *Miss Ugliness*.

Later, and with the new building, the helipad was relocated to the top of the parking structure.

Often times, the whole crew would be very busy with regular patients.

Whenever Air Rescue was making a drop, we would need to get an ER gurney out there on which to transfer the patient they were bringing in. John realized right away it was something I would be good at, since I could usually break away from my *really important* duty of rolling plastic, patient-garment bags.

And of course, I loved the variety in my work. Whenever we rushed a gurney out there, for safety's sake, we always had to wait until the rotors had completely stopped rotating before approaching.

Joseph Apple

I was puzzled after my first trip out there with two other nurses. There did not seem to be any big hurry with the female patient once we had her. This particular gal had fallen from a ladder and broken her arm while working on a log cabin out in the forest where an ambulance could not easily reach her.

We rolled her in with all the speed of delivering newspapers. I soon learned that the use of a helicopter was sometimes needed simply due to the remoteness of a location.

Sometimes it was urgent, and sometimes not.

One night, it was indeed an emergency as we grabbed our gurney.

John had instructed me to always remove the mattress pad before heading out there to prevent prop-wash from blowing it away. We were to roll the gurney to the top level, secure it next to the chain link fence, sit on the concrete steps just below the level of the landing pad...and then keep our heads down low.

At first, I thought they were being over-cautious...until my first copter landed.

Everyone should have to sit beneath a hovering helicopter to experience the tremendous force of air from the blades. I was duly impressed.

Our patient had been hunting in a wooded area and suffered a gunshot wound to his chest from a twelve-gauge shotgun. I was expecting the worst, since this would be my first time to be involved with a shotgun blast.

Dad had a couple of twelve-gauge shotguns in a closet downstairs which we would use when hunting rabbits in Indiana on Thanksgiving Day. We always went rabbit hunting on Thanksgiving Day.

I had witnessed what a 12-gauge shotgun could do to a rabbit up close and was not expecting this to be pretty.

I was there to help push the gurney and help with the heavy lifting...which I could do. We rushed the patient inside and to the trauma room.

As the ER surgeon removed the dressing applied by the air medics, I was surprised by what I saw. Instead of a neat hole being blown completely through the guy, as I usually saw on Daffy Duck cartoons, there was only a neat patch of exposed intestines on this guy's abdomen. My common sense told me it had to be bad.

The surgeon was in a hurry, but probed his forceps into the wound and withdrew a piece of *wadding* from the shotgun shell. I knew what was inside a shell after taking one apart as a kid to get at the gunpowder. I made the mistake of showing the powder to Dad, who yelled at me and told me to never do it again.

But with *wadding* stuck in the wound, I knew this had to have happened at very close range. I also did not give this guy much hope.

My brother Mike had once *unloaded* on a rabbit right in front of us while I had opted to let it get a little further away. I wanted enough of the rabbit to survive so we could have a *meal.* Actually, it was not that bad. The blast had blown away the entire belly of the rabbit...all the parts we would have not used anyway.

But to complicate the whole matter of this being an emergency, the air surgeon announced the wound was *self-inflicted.* He had done this to himself. And he was still alive!

I had seen on soap operas where an actor would get shot at point-blank range with a shotgun like this...maybe *two or three* times, and still live to talk about it in future episodes.

I did not believe it possible in *real life,* but I was looking at proof that it could indeed happen. At least, he was alive for the moment.

He was rapidly transported upstairs to OR for surgery where he may have died on the table. Personally, I doubt he pulled through. But it could have happened.

Joseph Apple

The thing that bothered me about the whole incident was all the waste when the guy had done it to himself. A helicopter had been rushed to him with highly-trained medical personnel, and then flown in risky conditions to a hospital where more highly-trained doctors, nurses and surgeons would work to save this guy's life...and for what?

If he recovered, there was a good chance he might try it again.

I was puzzled by it all.

It just did not seem right.

Equally puzzling was all the healing work performed on people wounded while committing acts of crime. It seemed to me that they had chosen their circumstances once they had decided to commit mayhem against another person.

In my *perfect world,* I would have all the guilty guys be worked on by medical students for practice. Then, all the innocent folk could get the good care.

I thought maybe it was a shame a person did not turn a certain **color** the instant they were involved in an incident that required medical attention.

I would have all the law offenders who had used a weapon during their crime turn a shade of dark brown, or black.

All those who had injected illegal drugs could turn purple.

All the drinking drivers could turn a shade of bright yellow.

All those who were innocent victims could turn a nice shade of light blue.

And all the bank robbers would turn bright red...something already done when a dye pack might explode in a money bag.

I might need to invent a few new shades to cover all the possibilities, but that's the way I would do it in my *perfect world.*

I understand that all life is considered sacred. But when you witness it up close in a trauma room, it often does not make much sense.

Color my world, "confused."

THE VOLUNTEER
SCREWS UP

It pains me to talk about this, but I'm not perfect.

One night I screwed up...and screwed up, *big time.*

Nothing happened as a result, but it could have been really bad.

I had spent several minutes with this old, ancient gal and her husband. I never learned why she was there, but she seemed to be improved from whatever had brought her to the ER that night.

She was to be discharged, and was sitting in a wheelchair waiting on paperwork. I had been away, and wanted to say goodbye before they took off. So I placed one hand on her right shoulder as a parting gesture.

Immediately, she said,

"Ohhhh, that feels so good!"

So I placed my other hand on the other shoulder and pressed equally as firmly with that hand as well. She moaned even more as to how good it felt.

Her husband was sitting on a chair next to us.

As I squeezed her shoulders, he remarked how he often rubbed her shoulders for her and said she really liked it when he would also squeeze the back of her neck. So, at his direction, I massaged the muscles along the sides of her spine in back of her neck.

She was loving all of this and moaning with pleasure in response to my touch.

When growing up with five sisters and four brothers, we would often rub each other's backs. And I was always quite good at it. I had perfected my sense of *feel* for tight muscles through my fingertips. I was proud of myself for the way I could rub a back and relieve a person's tension.

But while I was applying my method of *massage therapy*, I was aware that this gal's nurse, old *Punch Bag,* had stepped behind the counter and was placing a phone call.

Punch Bag was not like all the other nurses. She reminded me of the character on Saturday Night Live they all referred to as, "Pat."

"Is it a *he?*... is it a *she?*...we don't know. It's just, *Pat.*"

Pat looked like a gym punching bag with a *butch* haircut.

Pat also had the personality of a rabid Tasmanian devil. More than once, I had stepped in to comfort a patient after *he/she* had run roughshod over them.

Whenever *he/she* would instruct a patient to get out of their clothes and into a hospital gown, it often sounded like *he/she* was robbing them at gunpoint...

"*and put all your valuables in the bag!*"

My *spidy-sense* was tingling and the hairs on the back of my neck were standing on end.

So I ended the *massage session* and stepped to one side as we waited. After only a few seconds, the ER doctor appeared from around the corner and walked over to us. He just stood there and glared in my direction.

The old gal in the wheelchair mentioned how I had been giving her such a wonderful shoulder massage.

He stared at me with *hard* eyes and said,

"Yes...*so I heard.*"

I felt like a bank's *walk-in safe* where Lois Lane was trapped and Superman was using his blowtorch-vision to cut through the metal.

I am not a huge man, but I stand six feet tall. However, you could have measured my height with a six-inch ruler just then.

He didn't even speak to me, or otherwise acknowledge my presence. I felt like a trashcan, and he had just spit in it.

As he addressed his parting comments to his patient, I decided to slink on out of the room...like sludge creeping along a drainage ditch. I wanted to get far away from all of this. I had not felt like this in a long, long time...if *ever*.

Maybe the closest time was when I was thirteen and Dad had decided to cut my hair with his barber clippers the same way he had done when I was a little kid. I stayed in bed for three days before my wise mom took me to the barbershop for a *salvage* operation.

It was getting close to midnight, so I quickly made my way to the time clock and punched out. I only wanted to hurry to my car and get away from there.

I hoped to never run into that doctor ever again.

I am certain I never spoke to him again.

I know he was a good ER doctor after observing him work. But from that point on, I did not want to have anything more to do with him. I wished he had just *told me* to not do that again instead of treating me like a diseased leper.

But after thinking about it for several days, I realized he was right.

I did not agree with his method, but he was indeed right.

What he did not know was that I knew better than to massage any vascular areas on the gal. I was also being directed by the old gal's husband as I rubbed her shoulders. I had slid into it very easily.

But still, what I had done was wrong.

If the old gal had developed any problems at all, no matter what, the doctor and hospital could have been held responsible. And I would have been the scourge of society from that point on. It could have turned out very badly for everyone.

One of the things that made this even more difficult was the fact that John often used me in caring for his patients. But the difference this time was that I had acted on my own and not on the orders of someone in authority over me. That was my big mistake.

Some mistakes are painful enough that you don't need to worry about ever repeating them...like the time I stuck my tongue to the frosted trunk lid of Dad's '54 Pontiac.

After leaving *half* my tongue behind, I can safely say I will never repeat that act.

From then on, whenever I, the volunteer, was tempted to act on my own authority in the ER, I would rub the tip of my tongue against the backs of my front teeth...

...and *remember*.

REPEAT CUSTOMERS

I t was a slow night and I had all my obligations under control.

But still, I did not dare sit around. Dad had taught me to never *sit* when work was slow. He instructed me to first look for a broom and start sweeping...*slowly.*

He said to not go *too* fast, because I might be doing it for a while until things picked up. His point was to always *look* busy.

Pushing a broom was not an option in the ER since that was a job for Housekeeping only. Instead, I would sometimes grab a blanket or towel, place over one arm and walk rapidly along the halls.

I hate to admit this, but a couple of times I carried a blank sheet of paper in one hand as I walked briskly around the ER department....with a *frown* on my face.

It was a tricky job. I was most useful by being close by so the staff could grab me to do whatever was needed. But it would not look good if I just sat...and I knew that. I had overheard some of the staff complain about *other* volunteers who might sit around, reading a book.

I fully understood their dilemma because the ER was a scary place for a volunteer to work. Everyone was usually too busy to show you what to do.

You were just supposed to *know* what to do. You were also expected to somehow *magically* be right there…wherever you might be needed. It was an impossible task to satisfy everyone.

At first, I felt like a Christian in Roman times where you might get tossed into the arena with the lions. You had to somehow survive, and then return the following weekend to do it all again. It was a scary job.

One Saturday night, a nurse stopped me and said *my name* had come up in their weekly staff meeting. Someone had asked how the *volunteers* were working out in the ER, and several said they really liked the way *I* was performing my duties and that it would be great if they *all* would copy the way I did things.

I was very surprised to hear that since half the time I had little idea what I was doing. I guess no one in the department had ever read Hemingway's quote:

"Never mistake *movement* for *action*."

Sometimes, I was just *moving*.

But on Saturday nights, it usually was not long before someone would be rolled into the trauma room.

I strolled on in to the trauma room, opened the lower drawer of the center cabinet and placed booties over both shoes. It was not cool to track blood into the hallway.

A 40's Philippine male was rushed in with a self-inflicted knife wound to the chest.

We were all expecting the worst. As the surgeon removed the gauze dressing applied by paramedics, the patient was crying aloud, asking if he was going to die?

For the moment, I stood to one side as an observer.

The trauma surgeon probed the wound with an over-sized Q-tip.

I then noticed a rapid change in the surgeon's attitude as he realized this was no more than a minor flesh wound. The steak knife had only grazed the side of his rib cage and not done much damage.

The wound was not bad enough to require stitching, so the surgeon used surgical tape to close it up. He soon disposed of his gloves and was down the hallway and out of sight.

The patient then looked over to me as our eyes met. He asked *me* if he was going to live? So at this point, I stepped in and held his hand. He really gripped my hand hard, and I sensed he was in need of comfort. So I leaned over and got down on his level as I did my best to console him.

He began sharing with me all of his problems at home, and how he had lost his job. I had heard this story many times before, but it was all a brand new experience to this guy.

He confided to me that he had diabetes and some other problems that made him feel like a failure at home, and to his family. And I had to admit, he did have some problems. I kept hold of his hand and told him how things could improve and that there were services available to help him out.

I held his hand, patted him on the back and gave him lots of personal attention...which seemed to do the most good just then. I finally stepped aside to let the nurses finish dressing his wound.

I moved on, and I suppose he was sent home that night.

But the following Saturday night, a nurse came to me to share that *my friend* from last week was back in the trauma room *again* and asking for *me!* She said she did not know what I had done, but it must have been pretty good to get a *repeat customer*.

I was in the middle of changing out oxygen bottles on gurneys just then and could not go looking for him. But I did search for him as soon as I had the time. I suppose it was best that I missed him as he was carted off to County Mental Health.

I was quite impressed to have gotten a repeat customer asking for me specifically. I can understand requesting a favorite waitress at your local Steak and Shake.

But it was getting a little creepy when a guy was willing to jam a steak knife into his rib cage just to get *me!*

I suppose the best medicine for some people is to have a good friend, or mate available to hold their hand and just listen. Hospital emergency departments might be less crowded if this service was performed more often. A person doesn't even have to provide answers to be useful. You just need to get down on their level and dangle some *hope* in front of their eyes.

Oh, and you might want to also hide the steak knives.

DRUGS, SUICIDE AND OTHER FUN THINGS

My evening shift was over and I was talking with my good friend, Bob, the night security guy. He never said much, but we had become friends over the years.

I would often see him leaning against a wall somewhere trying to keep his eyes open. But that was the nature of his sort of work... seven hours and forty-five minutes of sheer boredom interrupted by fifteen minutes of life-threatening mayhem.

As we talked out on the sidewalk, a car pulled up with four occupants. They looked like a family on vacation stopping to ask directions. The mom and dad were in front of the black BMW sedan with two teenagers in the back seat.

The dad quickly jumped out of his seat and opened the rear door, revealing a teenage gal slumped against the door. The girls looked like they might have been sisters.

But the gal who was slumped over looked like she was totally out of it and unconscious. She was very pretty with long brunette hair, and dressed in a purple and off-white, floral silk bathrobe.

Once in a while this would happen...a *drop off*.

There would be no advance notice whatsoever...the patient

would just be dropped off and the staff would have to give it their best shot from there.

Bob ran inside and grabbed a wheelchair as the dad and I began pulling her out.

She felt almost lifeless as we got her into the chair. Once inside, the triage nurse began talking to her in a rough manner to get her attention. But that stopped once she realized this gal was really out of it.

They suspected the gal had taken some sort of drug, but no one knew what, or how much? This was typical with a drug overdose.

Often, no one would know exactly what had happened, and the ones who **did** know, would not want to talk. But the young gal's life would hinge on learning something about what had happened.

Sometimes, the cause for the emergency was a truly legitimate medical problem...but what? I learned later they pumped her stomach and gave her something to dilute the suspected chemicals she had ingested. But it sometimes did not go this well. She was a beautiful young lady and I hated to see this waste of youth.

One of the ER doctors confided to me that this sort of thing was one of the most challenging events for him. He would have to start from *scratch* and give it his best guess.

I hope she got help and never had this happen again.

On another night, I was hanging out with Nurse John and measuring the urine output from his patient. This job could be a little tricky if you did not do it just right. The patient would have a catheter inserted into their bladder and a long tube that emptied into a bag hanging on the side of the gurney.

I would have to open the valve on the bag and let it drain into a graduated cylinder. My first time to ever do this was on an over-filled bag that was about ready to burst.

Draining that bag was like trying to drain Hoover Dam with a garden hose hooked in at the base. Urine squirted out all over the place...and onto my arm...*yuck!* Fortunately, my task was simply to empty it and not gather a measurement.

John was having trouble with this patient. He had been sent over from a nursing home after ingesting a bottle of pills of some sort. He did not know exactly what? Our 80's patient had tried to end his life and was refusing to communicate with us. We knew he was awake, but he was not about to say anything.

John was trying to insert a naso-gastric tube into this guy's nose and on down into his stomach. But he could not get the tube past his throat. He had lubricated the tube and sprayed a numbing spray into his throat, but the thing was just not going.

After three failed attempts, he asked if I wanted to give it a shot? We were doing it together, so I wasn't doing anything all on my own.

Had I been doing it by myself, I would have removed the hose completely and straightened the tube a bit. After shining a light into his throat, I could tell that the hose was curling into a ball and not even getting past the back of his tongue.

In any event, I was not doing any better than John.

I knew the old dude was awake but pretending to be asleep. When we would ask him to open his mouth, he would do so. But he was not about to open his eyes or say anything.

It was a mess and nothing was working properly. And that was just the way things often went after a person had tried to commit suicide. Even the attempts to save the person often would not go well.

The ER doctor finally intervened and decided to go with a different procedure. I was called out and never learned what they did.

I leaned over the guy, patted his shoulder and said some things into his ear about how badly I felt for him. But there was nothing more I could do. I was very limited in what I had to offer in the first place. I really wanted to help him, but it was all just a big mess.

I always hoped his story turned out better than what I was seeing just then.

On yet another night, I went from bed-to-bed to see who might need some help.

As I poked my head into this one guy's cubicle, he yelled at me and began telling me how badly he was feeling and how his nurse would not come. He wanted a glass of water. I tracked down his nurse and asked if that would be okay...which it was. So I got him a glass of water with ice.

Getting water for a patient is not as simple as it might sound, since it could be very bad for a patient with an intestinal problem.

But this guy was grateful for my help. Amazingly, his demeanor changed abruptly in only a matter of five minutes after getting the water. He seemed to be an educated man and about the same age as myself.

So far, I had no idea why he was here.

In my volunteer training, we were advised to not share personal information with patients. But I found that impossible to follow.

Many of the patients wanted to talk, but did not yet know they wanted to talk.

If that sounds crazy...it probably is.

I knew from experience most patients would feel better if we could exchange information and I could let them know they were not alone in their struggle.

When I was a kid in Indiana, we had a water well just outside the back of the house. On top of the hand-dug well was a concrete slab with an iron hand-pump. I would have to crank on the pump handle to get any water out. But most of the time, nothing would come out without first *priming* the pump.

To *prime* a pump, I would need to first pour water in the top of the pump housing to cover the reed valves deep inside the well that were sucking air. And I could get into trouble if I forgot to fill the water bucket sitting at the base of the pump for the next guy after I was finished.

And this was my way of helping patients. I felt I needed to pour some of myself into them so they could get started on getting their own things out.

This guy had lots of stuff down inside him he wanted to get out, but just couldn't get it going. I was only doing with him what I did with everyone else in sharing pieces of my own life.

And that was all it took to get him going.

He began talking about how he had a successful home remodeling business.

Our present poor economy had hit him hard and he was having to watch his business fall apart all around him. He had to lay off most of the help and do all the paperwork himself.

He was really *gushing* now.

His whole lifestyle was taking a huge hit and his wife had just left him.

I finally realized he was in the ER because he had tried to take his own life.

He did not share with me exactly what he had done, and it was none of my business. But he made it clear he was having his problems.

I had plenty of experience with depression and shared some of my own details, which seemed to be of help to him. We talked for almost two hours that night and could have become good friends in any other type of situation. We had a lot in common and he seemed to be a really nice guy.

Eventually, *CMH* was there to take him to their facility.

I remember trying out for the football team when I was in the eighth grade.

Our school already had a really good football team because a bunch of the guys were not real smart and had flunked several grades. They should have been in high school already, and were **huge**.

The coach wanted to try me at **tight end.** But I did not yet have a helmet. Just then, the starting halfback threw me his very own helmet and told me to get on out there.

I was on cloud nine.

I had not yet entered into my growth spurt and was still one of the *little guys,* and did not make the team. But I will never forget that gesture from the starting halfback.

I am not sure if it is the same, but I feel like I am being of use if I can get down in the dirt with someone and let them know they are not alone in what they are experiencing.

Things can get pretty lonely when you are crawling around in the bottom of a deep, dark hole.

I did not have a helmet to loan him, but figured maybe I could be of help by throwing part of myself out there.

I don't know how much I really helped that guy in the long run, but I know for sure he was feeling better when I left. I hope he was able to get his life turned around.

HERE COME THE
CLOWNS

The emergency room on a Saturday night often looked some sort of *costume ball* with the way patients would be dressed.

One patient might be in ragged jeans while the next could be in a tuxedo. People came in from whatever they happened to be doing that Saturday night.

I remember one patient dressed in a black tuxedo who had passed out at a bachelor party. The paramedics said they found him unconscious on the ballroom floor of a hotel after he had rapidly downed a whole bottle of vodka.

Many people seem to be in denial about alcohol being a drug. But that's what it is....a **drug**, *ethyl alcohol.*

The only reason it is not considered a poison is because human blood contains the necessary enzymes to break the stuff down to get rid of it...dehydrogenase, alcohol dehydrogenase, cytochrome p-450 and a couple of others.

Methyl and *Propyl* alcohol are also regular alcohols, but our blood cannot break them down...and thus they will kill a person who is stupid enough to drink them.

Alcohol takes its toll on a body by causing liver scarring from the intermediate by-product, acetaldehyde. When alcohol is ingested in excess, the body will dump its electrolytes, causing the *sodium/potassium* pump to fail.

The bottom line is, your heart can stop...*dead.*

Throughout the entire night, our tuxedo-drunk never did regain consciousness. All the staff who were caring for him brought others in to look at him...*the guy who could not hold his liquor.*

Half the male staff confessed to having been in a similar situation at some time in their past, and they all thought it was rather funny.

The guy almost died right there and they had to rig his body up with some special heated pads to help control his body temperature.

The nurses decided to pull a prank on the guy after finding his cell phone. They took his photo with all the tubes and IV's running into him and placed that photo on his phone as his *screen saver.* And I suppose it was a good idea for the guy to know how he looked.

I thought it was unfortunate the patient was missing out on the whole ordeal by being unconscious. Hopefully he would learn some day that you don't have to get *wasted* in order to have a good time.

But then again, he may never get it.

We all are fragile human beings in need of care. Some of us live careful lives while others seem to throw caution to the wind each day...for whatever reason.

In the ER, I did my best to help people who were having a worse day than myself, but sometimes felt like I was working the center ring of Barnum and Bailey.

Joseph Apple

So bring on the clowns...

...but beware of the lions.

www.ingramcontent.com/pod-product-compliance
Lightning Source LLC
Chambersburg PA
CBHW021820170526
45157CB00007B/2663